Conflict, peace and mental health

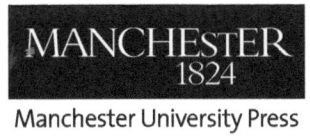

Conflict, peace and mental health

Addressing the consequences of conflict and trauma in Northern Ireland

DAVID BOLTON

Manchester University Press

Copyright © David Bolton 2017

The right of David Bolton to be identified as the author of this work has been asserted by him in accordance with the Copyright, Designs and Patents Act 1988.

Published by Manchester University Press
Altrincham Street, Manchester M1 7JA

www.manchesteruniversitypress.co.uk

British Library Cataloguing-in-Publication Data
A catalogue record for this book is available from the British Library

ISBN 978 0 7190 9099 8 hardback
ISBN 978 1 5261 2667 2 paperback

First published 2017

Reprinted 2018

The publisher has no responsibility for the persistence or accuracy of URLs for any external or third-party internet websites referred to in this book, and does not guarantee that any content on such websites is, or will remain, accurate or appropriate.

Typeset in 10.5/12.5 Adobe Garamond by
Servis Filmsetting Ltd, Stockport, Cheshire
Printed in Great Britain by
CPI Group (UK) Ltd, Croydon CR0 4YY

Dedicated to the people of Enniskillen and the people of Omagh, who held together in times that might otherwise have driven them apart.

Contents

List of figures and tables viii
List of abbreviations and glossary ix
Acknowledgements xii
Timeline xviii

Introduction 1
1 The Omagh bombing and the community's response 8
2 The Omagh Community Trauma and Recovery Team 25
3 Assessing the mental health impact of the Omagh bombing 39
4 The mental health impact of the Troubles, 1969–1999 53
5 The mental health impact of the Troubles, 2000–2015 70
6 The Northern Ireland Centre for Trauma and Transformation: a comprehensive trauma centre 103
7 The development of a trauma-focused therapy programme 117
8 Trauma-focused skills training for practitioners 138
9 Research, advocacy and policy support 151
10 Planning for and responding to the mental health impact of conflict 169
Postscript: the rupture of loss and trauma 186

Bibliography 190
Index 203

Figures and tables

Figures

1. Illustration of the pattern of referrals to the Omagh Community Trauma and Recovery Team, over two-and-a-half years, from August 1998.   34
2. Illustration of the PDS and GHQ caseness levels for adults, for each type of exposure to the Omagh Bombing (Duffy et al., 2013).   43
3. Illustration of the mean PTSD and stress scores of staff involved in the response to the Omagh bombing, compared with scores for those who were not involved (Luce et al., 2003).   50
4. Number of self-help groups formed in Northern Ireland in relation to the Belfast Agreement (From Dillenburger et al., 2006).   68
5. A needs-led and trauma-focused public health framework for service development and building workforce capability in communities affected by long-term stressors.   142
6. The prevalence of lifetime mental health disorders in the Northern Ireland Study of Health and Stress across three trauma categories (Bunting et al., 2012).   159
7. Overview of possible measures to promote the capabilities of community members and key services to address the immediate and long-term impact of major traumatic stressors on individuals, families and communities.   176

Tables

1. Framework for considering the impact of community tragedies (Bolton, 1999).   13
2. Overview of the NICTT's integrated trauma-focused workforce development framework.   147
3. An example of a competence framework developed by the NICTT, outlining core competences of workers operating in key parts of a trauma stepped-care system.   183

Abbreviations and glossary

CBT	cognitive behavioural therapy – one of a number of psycho-social interventions combining behavioural and cognitive approaches to counselling or therapy, which is underpinned by a distinctive set of principles and practices, and an extensive evidence base.
DHSS	Department of Health and Social Services – Northern Ireland's health and social care department up until 1999.
DHSSPS	Department of Health and Social Services and Public Safety – the abbreviation used from 1999 until 2016 to refer to Northern Ireland's health and social care department.
loyalism	A term used to refer to the political movement that promotes the union of Northern Ireland with Britain. The term is often used interchangeably with 'unionism'.
nationalism	A term used to refer to the political movement that aspires to a unified and autonomous Ireland. The term is often used interchangeably with 'republicanism'.
NICE	National Institute for Health and Care Excellence – develops and publishes guidance on health technologies, health practice, health promotion and guidance relating to social care. Its remit relates to the National Health Service in England and Wales. Originally known as the National Institute for Clinical Excellence (1999–2005).
NICTT	Northern Ireland Centre for Trauma and Transformation (2002–2011) – established to develop and deliver a programme for the treatment of trauma-related disorders related to the Troubles. Based in Omagh, the Centre also had programmes for research, training and education, policy and advocacy, and humanitarian relief.
NISHS	Northern Ireland Study of Health and Stress – undertaken by the Ulster University in 2005–2008 as one the World Mental Health Survey Initiative series of national studies. The NISHS

	was funded by the Research and Development Office of Northern Ireland's health department.
OFMDFM	Office of the First Minister and Deputy First Minister – the central administrative department of Northern Ireland governing Executive. The term was used from 1999 until 2016.
paramilitaries	The term widely used in Northern Ireland to refer to non-state armed groups.
psycho-social	An approach to the physical and mental well-being of individuals that seeks to promote wellness and functioning through an understanding of their psychological difficulties and strengths, along with an understanding of their family and other relationships, and their social and economic circumstances.
PTSD	post-traumatic stress disorder – a specific psychological disorder which includes as one of its essential criteria that a person must have had a traumatic experience. This means the concept is particularly useful for understanding and responding to the needs of people who have been affected by life threatening or other traumatic experiences, as well as understanding the impact of commonly experienced stressors (such as those caused by war and violent conflict) on populations.
republicanism	A term used to refer to the political movement that aspires to a unified and autonomous Ireland. The term is often used interchangeably with 'nationalism'.
SEUPB	Special European Union Programme Body: the body established in 1995 following the ceasefires by armed groups and which later became one of six cross-border bodies – subsequent to the Belfast Agreement of 1998. The role of the SEUPB was to manage cross-border European Union Structural Funds programmes in Northern Ireland, the Border Region of Ireland and parts of western Scotland. Its programmes included PEACE I, II, II and IV, which were made available by EU donors with additional funding from the British and Irish Governments, along with other European Structural Funds such as Interreg I, II, III and IV.
the Troubles	The term widely used in Northern Ireland to refer to the period of civil conflict that is generally agreed to have commenced in 1969. Some consider the year of the Belfast Agreement (1998) to be the end of the Troubles. Since the Agreement, the general level of violence has reduced

	considerably. However, others, noting that people have been killed and otherwise seriously affected by violence since the Agreement, take the view that the end of the Troubles has not yet been reached (i.e. by 2017).
UU	The Ulster University (previously known as the University of Ulster).
unionism	A term used to refer to the political movement that promotes the union of Northern Ireland with Britain. The term is often used interchangeably with 'loyalism'.

Acknowledgements

What follows reflects the concerns and efforts of many, not just one person. I wish to record and acknowledge the contribution to this work of those who have suffered loss, injury and trauma over the course of nearly thirty years and whom I have met along the way. On nearly every page, a child, a parent, an adult or a family came to mind as I wrote. Their loss, suffering, realities, insights and hopes, their sometimes arresting view of things, pervade the thoughts and purposes behind this book. Likewise, I wish to record and acknowledge the contributions of the hundreds of individuals whose lives touched mine and whose efforts brought consolation, support and healing to those who have suffered – from the passing act of neighbourly kindness that made all the difference, to the life given over to this work. I remember especially the humanitarian efforts of manager, practitioner and administrator colleagues whose compassion, skill and professionalism I was privileged to witness at first hand on many occasions. Similarly, across Northern Ireland, throughout the Troubles, many individuals, services and communities provided what support they could – often in the most difficult of circumstances. My experience has been that in the deepest adversity the best of humanity can be found. The collective generosity of those who suffered and the efforts of those who sought to help them stand over and against the worst that we can do to each other. Beauty, instead of ashes.

Services such as those developed in Omagh following the bombing and later in the work of the Northern Ireland Centre for Trauma and Transformation (NICTT) could not have been established or sustained without the support of funders. Many funders and donors – public, charitable, private and personal – have contributed to the body of work described in the following pages. I gratefully acknowledge the contribution of: the Sperrin Lakeland Trust; the Northern Ireland Office (NIO), the Omagh Fund, the European Union's PEACE II and Interreg funds and Cooperating and Working Together (CAWT), the UK's Big Lottery Fund, Northern Ireland's Executive Office (formerly the Office of the First Minister and Deputy First Minister), the Lupina Foundation, The Atlantic Philanthropies, Northern Ireland's Department of Health (formerly the Department of Health, Social Services and Public Safety), the Community

Acknowledgements

Relations Council and other funders. Appreciation also to the Special European Union Programme Body (SEUPB), which managed the European Union's Programme for Peace and Reconcilliation, for its interest in the research and work of the NICTT. The support interest and encouragement of those individuals in funding bodies, who were motivated by their concern for those in need and their desire to see good things happen, is not forgotten.

When so many have played a part, thanking and acknowledging are fraught with the problem of adequately reflecting whose contribution should be acknowledged. So, mindful of the support and friendship of many, there are some I would like to thank in particular for their companionship and collegiality along the way. First, from the earlier days, I think of my boss at the time, Freda Carson, who along with two local teachers Kate Doherty and Toni Johnston with courage, concern, intuitive caring and commitment, did so much to bring support to children, adults and families affected by the Enniskillen bombing (Doherty, 1991). In 1989, following the Kegworth aircrash, Marion Gibson and I worked together representing Northern Ireland's Health and Social Services in the East Midlands, England. Marion has contributed much to the development of practice in the wake of disasters, in Northern Ireland and elsewhere. Then, from our work in the aftermath of the Omagh bombing, I remember in particular, Hugh Mills, chief executive, and Richard Scott, chairman, of the local public health and social care services agency, the Sperrin Lakeland Health and Social Care Trust, whose intuitive and enabling leadership at a time of great crisis for our organisation, made good things happen – including the establishment of the Omagh Community Trauma and Recovery Team. I recall the tireless work of fellow directors, senior managers, practitioners and administration colleagues as we sought to bring order out of the chaos of the immediate aftermath and in the long term ensure services were available to the community. I remember vividly those I worked alongside in the hours and days following the bombing, colleagues from my own organisation – the Sperrin Lakeland Trust – and those from other organisations and places who volunteered to work alongside us. I recall too the wider community of those who worked to bring help and support, including members of the public, neighbours and friends, colleagues from local not-for-profit agencies, the clergy and leaders from local churches and faith communities, the family liaison officers from the local police service, and the staff at Omagh Leisure Centre, who made a significant contribution to the practical care of those who needed it. And there was the important work of colleagues who kept services going for those who had not been affected by the bombing, yet still required medical, nursing, social care and other services.

From the early days of our work in Omagh following the bombing in 1998, Kate Gillespie, consultant psychiatrist and accomplished cognitive therapist, contributed greatly to the development of the trauma therapy service, and through her skill and commitment helped so many along the way. Michael

Duffy, experienced social worker and skilled cognitive therapist who, with a detailed knowledge of Omagh and the wider community, energetically coordinated the work of the Omagh Team for over three years and who likewise did much to help people through his therapeutic work. Kate and Michael later contributed centrally to the development of the NICTT and in particular the provision of its therapy, research and education services. Key to progress was the commitment of many practitioners, including Sean Collins and colleagues from various disciplines who, following the bombing in 1998, formed the early team and in some cases contributed over many years, including with the NICTT. James Baxter and Michael Skuce, Omagh's senior police officers, Eddie Morton, Eddie Giboney and their colleagues worked closely with us to coordinate the support for individuals and families affected directly by the bombing. Maura McDermott, child and adolescent consultant psychiatrist, led the development of services for children and young people caught up in the explosion and was central to the study which assessed their needs in the aftermath. Clive Burges, occupational health consultant, played a key role in the development of services to support the staff of the local hospitals and community services who had responded to the bombing and was instrumental in the important study of staff needs in the years following the bombing. I remember too administration colleagues, especially the late James Johnston, Daphne Armstrong, Anne Donaghy and Esther Stewart and their colleagues, without whom we would have been lost and who brought much to the services of which they were an essential part. Colleagues in the local mental health services played a key role in supporting the local community and in volunteering for the trauma Team over the course of its lifetime. I recall the tireless contributions of the Reverend Robert Herron and Father Kevin Mullan who with other faith leaders contributed so much to the stability of the Omagh community, and whose liturgical and pastoral responses, along with their insights and support, helped us in the development of services. Joe Martin, chief executive of the local education authority, Jack Walls who was assigned to liaise between the schools and the Team, their colleagues, and local school principals and teachers, were key to establishing a relationship between the pivotal work of schools in support of children and the work of the Omagh Community Trauma and Recovery Team. The officers and politicians at Omagh District Council contributed much to the response and recovery of the local community, and I recall in particular the leadership of John McKinney, chief executive, the staff at the Leisure Centre under the leadership of Phillip Faithful, and the creative and enabling contribution of Frank Sweeney. The editors and staff of the two local newspapers, the *Tyrone Constitution* and the *Ulster Herald*, played such an important role in telling the wider world about the impact of the bombing and provided valuable information and support for local people.

Several academics contributed to the development of the strategic direction of services and to the understanding of the impact of the bombing on the community. David Clark, professor of psychiatry, Ann Hackmann, Freda McManus, Anke Ehlers and their colleagues at Oxford University were instrumental in the therapeutic approach at the heart of the therapy programme. With local services, they undertook the needs-assessment of adults within a year of the bombing, upon which later developments were founded. Similarly, Jenny Firth-Cozens of the University of Northumbria, and her colleagues Anna Luce and Simon Midgley helped us understand the impact of the bombing on health and social care staff and thereafter greatly influenced the development of staff care services. Andy Percy and the late Patrick McCrystal from Queens University Belfast, along with Michael Fitzgerald from Trinity College Dublin, collaborated with local practitioners to undertake the important needs-assessments of children and adolescents, which again influenced the development of services.

When the decision was taken some years after the Omagh bombing to establish the NICTT, it required the formation of a governing trust. The steadfast contribution of the trustees was central to the work of the Centre. I am profoundly grateful to the tireless leadership, wisdom and support of the chairman, Fabian Monds, who was originally from Omagh, with a background as an entrepreneur and leading academic. I also pay tribute to the other trustees, Brian Patterson (business leader), David McKittrick (journalist and writer, and co-author of an iconic chronicle of the deaths in the Troubles, *Lost Lives*), Paul Seawright (professor of photography and esteemed photographer of the Troubles), Roy McClelland (professor of mental health and co-chair and author of a major review of mental health needs and services in Northern Ireland – the Bamford Report – DHSSPS, 2007), Sacha, Duchess of Abercorn (from the Omagh area, practitioner in transformation and founder of The Pushkin Trust focusing on the developmental and educational potential of children), and Sinead McLaughlin (a primary school principal from Buncrana, Co. Donegal). They brought presence, along with highly relevant skills and experiences to their task. Together they have made a remarkable contribution of public service in the interests of those who have been adversely affected by the Troubles. They have provided the platform upon which services could be developed, in which pivotal research was undertaken, training developed and from which other communities in far away places that were affected by conflict, could be helped.

Others played pivotal roles in the development and work of the Centre. I recall the passionate concern of Sean O'Dwyer, chairman of the the Omagh Fund, whose encouragement, along with the support of the Fund's trustees and officer, Brian Oliphant, enabled the Centre to take hold in the imagination of those who sought to support adults, children and families affected by the bombing. The Fund's long view of and concern for the needs of those affected psychologically by the bombing was highly influential in shaping the work undertaken in response to the bombing, and later by the NICTT. My thanks to Hugh Mills, chief executive of the Sperrin Lakeland Trust, John McKinney, chief executive of Omagh District Council, Tom Frawley, chief executive of the Western Health and Social Services Board (the Sperrin Lakeland Trust's service commissioner) and John O'Neill and colleagues at Venture International, who were instrumental in early progress on the development of the Centre. And thanks also for the considerable support in the early days following the bombing in Omagh and in the years that followed, of John McFaul and Des Browne, Parliamentary Under-Secretaries of State (both of whom were subsequently appointed life peers in the UK House of Lords) and their colleagues at the NIO, with William Stevenson and Mary Lemon, civil servants at the NIO's Victims Liaison Unit in Belfast, for their interest, advice and support and for making funding available at a critical time. My thanks also to John Clarke at the Victims Unit (OFMDFM) for his interest and support especially in relation to the training and education work of NICTT.

My thanks to all our other colleagues at the NICTT, including Eileen MacMackin, Ruth Liggett, Tracey McCrossan, Gemma Rankin and other administration colleagues, whose contribution was at the heart of its work. Besides those already mentioned, the Centre's therapy team included Geraldine Kerr, who was the first point of contact for many who sought our help, and therapists Susan McGandy, John McLaren and Paul Quinn. In the later years, Brendan Armstrong, cognitive therapist and clinical director at the Centre brought much to the further development of its therapy and education services. Maria Kee, psychiatrist and cognitive therapist, brought innovative approaches to the delivery of training thereby helping many in non-clinical settings, and individuals and families affected by traumatic experiences. Our partnership with Brendan Bunting, principal investigator and professor of research psychology at the Ulster University, with Finola Ferry the lead researcher, Siobhan O'Neill and Sam Murphy, led to an extensive body of research over ten years, which examined the population impact of the Troubles and which came to form the definitive epidemiological assessment of the impact of the Troubles. The partnership was enabled by the Research and Development Division of Northern Ireland's Public Health Agency, with the interest and support of its former Director, Bernie Hannigan. Key research was funded by Peter Warrian and Margret Hovenec's Lupina Foundation which established an early interest in the work of the Centre and who, through a sustained relationship of interest and financial support, were also able to contribute to the Centre's work in support of other conflict-affected communities. Barney Devine who, as business manager of the Centre, not only believed passionately in the mission of the Centre but from his years in education, and in peace and reconciliation work in Northern Ireland, saw how addressing the mental health impact of the Troubles was a critical concern for peace-makers. For his enduring support and friendship, I am most grateful.

Acknowledgements

The book has been made possible by the encouragement, practical and kind support of the chairman and trustees of the NICTT Trust, by the Department of Foreign Affairs and Trade in Dublin, and with the help and assistance of the staff at Manchester University Press, to whom I express my appreciation. My thanks to Rachel Evans, copy-editor, for her careful and gracious handling of the text, and to Dominic Carroll, for his comprehensive index. My thanks also to those writers and researchers who willingly provided copies of research reports and papers, and who answered queries. I am thankful to David McKittrick and Hugh Mills for their careful proofreading of the text, and to them, David Clark, Barney Devine, Kate Doherty, Michael Duffy, Kate Gillespie, Robert Herron, Roy McClelland, Fabian Monds, Eddie Morton, Kevin Mullan, Sean O'Dwyer, Brian Oliphant and Richard Scott, for their observations and suggestions. I am grateful to Paul Seawright whose picture *Steps* is on the front cover, one of several we were privileged to have on the NICTT corporate literature over the years.

Finally, my wife Helen, our daughters – and in adulthood their growing families – have been an enduring source of strength, support and encouragement over the years. They have shared closely in some of the events described herein. This book is in many ways an account of their journey also. To Helen, Julie, Leah and Alison – my utmost respect and deepest appreciation.

Through this book I hope that something of the efforts of this *cast of many* will reach people we will never meet and places we will never visit, but with whom we share and express our concern, support and hope.

David Bolton, Enniskillen
January 2017

Timeline

Year	Events linked to the Troubles and the peace process	Events associated with this book
1969	The first major violence linked to the Troubles of the period 1969–1998	
1971	Serious violence in Belfast, Derry/Londonderry and elsewhere in Northern Ireland	
1972	Serious violence in Belfast, Derry/Londonderry and elsewhere in Northern Ireland Bloody Sunday; 14 killed by British Army soldiers – 30 January Bloody Friday; 9 killed by 20 IRA bombs across Belfast – 21 July	
1973	The Sunningdale Agreement – involving British and Irish Governments and pro-agreement parties – 9 December	
1974	Assembly and Executive formed in January; collapses in May after Ulster Workers Strike Dublin and Monaghan bombings; 34 killed – 17 May Birmingham bombings; 21 killed – 21 November	
1976	Formation of Peace People movement after deaths of three children in traffic collision linked to the Troubles	
1978	The La Mon Hotel firebombed; 12 killed – 17 February	
1979	Lord Mountbatten, family members and a boy from Enniskillen killed in bomb explosion on his boat near Sligo by IRA; on the same day 18 soldiers and a civilian killed near Warrenpoint – 27 August Pope John Paul visits Ireland and calls for an end to violence – September	

Timeline xix

Year	Events linked to the Troubles and the peace process	Events associated with this book
1980–81	The Hunger Strikes; ten republican prisoners die with significant street violence and political implications	
1983	New Ireland Forum announced and meets in Dublin – May	
1985	The Anglo-Irish Agreement – 15 November;	
1987		The Enniskillen Remembrance Sunday bombing – 8 November
1988	Humes-Adams round of talks begin (January) and end with no agreement (September)	
1990	Mary Robinson elected President of Ireland, assuming office on 3 December	
1991	IRA attack 10 Downing Street, London – 7 February	
1992	Bombing of workers van at Teebane; 8 killed – 17 January Shooting at Bookmaker's shop in Belfast; 5 killed – 5 February President Clinton lifts USA visa ban for Gerry Adams — April	
1993	Joint Declaration on Peace (The Downing Street Declaration) – 15 December	
1994	IRA ceasefire, 31 August Loyalist armed groups ceasefire – 13 October	
1996	IRA ceasefire ends – 9 February	
1997	IRA ceasefire reinstated – 20 July	
1998	The Belfast Agreement (The Good Friday Agreement) – 10 April Referendums north and south support the Belfast Agreement – 22 May First Victims Commissioner's Report published – May	The Omagh bombing – 15 August The Omagh Community Trauma and Recovery Team is established
1999–2000		Four major needs assessments of the impact of the Omagh bombing undertaken

Year	Events linked to the Troubles and the peace process	Events associated with this book
2001	New Police Service of Northern Ireland formed – 4 November	The Omagh Community Trauma and Recovery Team closes – June
2002		The Northern Ireland Centre for Trauma and Transformation opens – May
2003		NICTT-UU research partnership formed
2004	The Leeds Castle talks end with no agreement	
2006	The St Andrews Agreement – 13 October Legislation put in place for the Victims and Survivors Commission and other structures (Victims and Survivors (Northern Ireland) Order, 2006)	
2007	Interim Victims and Survivors Commissioner's Report published	
2008	Amending legislation put in place for Commission for Victims and Survivors; four commissioners appointed	Trauma, Health and Conflict Report – first report from NICTT-UU research partnership with estimates of the population impact on mental health of the Troubles
2009	Consultative Group on the Past publishes its report – 28 January	
2010	The Saville Enquiry into Bloody Sunday published – 15 June	

Year	Events linked to the Troubles and the peace process	Events associated with this book
2011		Police officer killed when bomb in his car explodes in Omagh – 2 April The Northern Ireland Centre for Trauma and Transformation closes – 31 December
2012	Comprehensive Needs Assessment report published by the Commission for Victims and Survivors (CVSNI, 2012)	
2013	The Haass-O'Sullivan interparty talks end in no agreement – 31 December	
2014	The Stormont House Agreement – 23 December – which later collapsed in 2015	
2015	Health minister announces plans to establish a trauma mental health service – 11 September The Fresh Start Agreement – 17 November	
2016	Funding announcement for new trauma mental health service – 24 February	
2017	Northern Ireland Assembly and Executive collapse and elections called – 16 January	

With thanks to McKittrick and McVea (2012).

Introduction

Two days after a car bomb exploded in the town of Omagh in Northern Ireland on 15 August 1998, the British Secretary of State for Northern Ireland, the late Dr Marjorie Mowlam M.P., visited the town. In the context of a terrible atrocity her visit was both ceremonial and highly focused on the real risk the bombing posed for the recent peace agreement (the Belfast or Good Friday Agreement), which marked the culmination of talks between most of Northern Ireland's political parties and the British and Irish Governments. The Agreement, finalised on 10 April 1998, had raised hopes of a historic political settlement to the Troubles – the years of civil conflict in Northern Ireland that had commenced in 1969.

On the morning of Dr Mowlam's visit to Omagh, I was one of a small group of health and social care practitioners who had been involved in responding to the bombing, from shortly after the bomb exploded. When she arrived at the temporary trauma centre that had been hurriedly set up that morning, she wanted to hear about the consequences of the bombing for those directly affected and for the wider community. What I recall most clearly from our conversation were two incisive questions posed by the Secretary of State. What would the human impact of the bombing be? And what needed to be done to address that impact?

It has taken over fifteen years to provide competent answers to these important questions and it is from the experience of struggling with them that this book has emerged. It is hoped that for readers needing to know how best to address the mental health and related impacts of conflict on their communities, the book will be of interest and assistance, and a resource that they can return to time and again. By sharing experiences of addressing the conflict-related violence in Northern Ireland, I hope that readers can short-circuit such a long gestation period and be able to use the lessons and messages from the following pages to plan for and provide informed responses in the context of their own experiences. As a consequence I hope that those who suffer through violent conflict in places far from Northern Ireland, will benefit. Also, with the passing of time I felt it necessary to make some record of what was learnt through terrible events for the benefit of others, before memory fades.

During the Troubles and since, many services aimed at helping communities and individuals were established, funded and provided in response to the violence – many of which were supported by charitable, governmental or European funding. Further, long standing publicly provided mental health services and practitioners, and other health and social care staff, along with local and regional not-for-profit services and self-help groups, have in various ways sought to understand and address the impact of the Troubles, and to address the needs of individuals, families and communities. Often, these contributions and efforts held the line for individuals, families and communities, whilst politics struggled to address wider legacy issues, including services to those affected by the years of violence. This book offers and draws upon one account of that wider response to the Troubles. It will be relevant to mental health policy-makers, service planners, providers and practitioners. However, it is hoped that others will read it too, such as peace-makers, diplomats, politicians, civil servants and those who have engaged in violent conflict and war who are seeking to understand the impact of violence on their communities.

Across the world conflicts start, rage and end – leaving behind the most terrible of human tragedies and needs, shaped by loss and trauma. As they rage and after they end, individuals, families, communities, government departments and aid agencies are faced with the task of reconstruction, recovery and adjustment. Some individuals, however, cannot make the transition. One of the areas of need that threatens the long-term well-being and competence of the post-war or post-conflict community is the impact of violent conflict and war on the mental health of citizens and displaced persons. Whilst we can hope, even expect, most people will cope with and recover from terrible personal loss and traumatic experiences, we now know that in communities affected by conflict, war and disasters, a significant minority will have mental health and related problems in the short, medium and long term. We know too that the longer conflict rages and the more traumatic the experiences suffered by individuals and communities, the greater the proportion of the community that will suffer longer-term adverse consequences. We know this gives rise to major social and economic challenges for survivors and has intergenerational impact. The mental health and related consequences of conflict can limit engagement, participation and belonging in the emerging post-conflict community. Recognising and addressing the health and well-being impacts of violence is an important task in enabling as many as possible to become stakeholders in and contributors to the emerging post-conflict community. In the context of building peace there is therefore a wider interest in attending to the personal and family consequences of conflict.

The central message of this book, therefore, is that addressing the mental health and wider needs arising from loss and trauma must be incorporated as early as possible into the peace-making and peace-building project. In contemporary warfare and conflict the dead and surviving victims are increasingly civilians who had not been protagonists. They bear the greatest heat of the day, and their needs often fade rapidly from the minds of those who waged war and now make peace. In some sense it should be an easy thing to address – to provide for the needs of those who have suffered loss and trauma. It should be a quick win for the post-conflict politics, an expression of hope in the investment in peace. But it often does not seem so. Time and again victims and survivors are left behind. The experiences behind the writing of this book suggest at least three reasons for this problem.

First, other things seem to be more important – such as ceasefires, peace talks, constitutional settlements, the standing down of armies and armed groups, the establishment of institutions and political processes, economic investment, the demands for and trade-offs in justice, the recognition of minorities. The pressing daily needs of humanity are something we will get round to in due course.

There is another dynamic. Those who wage war, or are protagonists in civil conflict, and the politicians have to sit with mortal and ideological enemies and make peace. Painful and uncomfortable things have to be addressed or valued things set aside to allow progress. One of the discomfitures is the dead – my dead and your dead – along with those who mourn, those who have been injured, and those whose lives have been changed by the trauma of their experiences. I dare not press my case too hard, to remind you that you, or those with whom you allied yourself, caused my dead – because I will be reminded that the reverse may also be true. Or be reminded by my own community that the things for which the dead died, are no longer as important or centre stage as they once seemed to be. They have yielded to the necessity of bringing hostilities to an end and building peace. Add to this the continuing, often heated, battle over who is a victim and who deserves access to services, and the hopes of progress for those who have suffered can go unrealised. In Ireland, whilst the dead of our civil conflicts are held sacred by one side or another (seldom by all), the suffering survivors run the risk of being abandoned because we cannot politically agree on how they ought to be helped. Whilst the rest of the world moves on, those who are disabled by their experience of hostility, loss, injury or trauma are caught in an unsatisfactory present. Left in a liminal state – a no-man's land between the past and the emerging future with nowhere to go back to yet feeling unable to go forward – surviving victims of the conflict become, also, victims of the peace.

Finally, there is the difficulty in understanding the problem and therefore the solutions. Partly this is to do with the view that people suffering loss and trauma cannot be helped, or that if they are to overcome their experiences it is something that cannot be addressed by the peace-building project. Sometimes, it might be that there is no solution in the peace agreement for displaced people, who for example remain displaced, living far from home or in refugee camps. There can be a view that the answer to the deep psychological needs of those who suffer lies in justice and reparation. Or conversely, that there is purely a psychological solution to needs that, besides the experience of loss and trauma, have components of injustice, deprivation or victimhood and require political action. The challenge is to understand needs accurately without adopting ideological solutions. Asking people about their needs and views is an important starting point, and if necessary an on-going requirement as people's needs and views change. Getting the balance right between helping people to become increasingly members of, and stakeholders in, the emerging post-conflict community whilst attending properly and effectively to their need to heal and recover is of central importance. Certainly we should be mindful that locally, needs and solutions will differ, and will be determined by local priorities and realities. It is hoped that this book contributes to these considerations.

These experiences change us for ever

The Omagh bombing had striking resonances for me, with a similar bombing in Enniskillen, eleven years earlier, on 8 November 1987. Writing about the Enniskillen bombing in 1997, on the occasion of the tenth anniversary, McDaniel asked whether in the light of the awfulness of that atrocity 'such a dreadful thing could happen again' (McDaniel, 1997: 8). It did – and just a year after the question was posed – it happened in Omagh. In both towns, the circumstances involved a bomb exploding in a street where civilians had gathered: in Enniskillen for a ceremony of remembrance; in Omagh, for refuge after a bomb alert. In both circumstances I had been immediately and directly involved with colleagues in addressing the concerns and needs of those caught up in the bombings: assisting with the injured; supporting the emergency health services; helping people to find missing relatives; comforting the distressed; responding to enquiries from the media, and, most terrible of all, locating and identifying the dead.

There were differences in the two tragedies. Enniskillen had resulted in fewer deaths and injuries. In fact, the local hospital in Enniskillen had more seriously injured people admitted on the day of the Omagh bombing, than it had on the occasion of the Enniskillen bombing. By merit of the scale of those who were killed, injured and distressed, the Omagh bombing, it turned out, would become the largest single atrocity associated with the recent period of civil conflict in Northern Ireland. It impacted not only on Omagh and its hinterland of villages and rural neighbourhoods but also on people from Donegal (in the Republic of Ireland) and visitors from Madrid in Spain.

The Enniskillen bombing was perceived as an attack on one of Northern Ireland's traditions, whereas the Omagh bombing impacted upon individuals and families from across the cultural and political spectrum. Enniskillen happened when violence was still raging, when a political solution seemed impossible and when hope could take no concrete form in the imagination. Omagh came after the historic Belfast Agreement, after the main non-state armed groups had declared ceasefires and following demilitarisation by the British Army.

The Enniskillen bombing had considerable consequences for children and their schools and it was in this context mainly that I, along with colleagues, began some work with local teachers. Over the following ten years, that work involved trying to understand and respond to the grief and trauma-related needs of families and individuals alongside the contributions and efforts of neighbours, the wider community and its civil institutions, its schools and churches. By the time of the Omagh bombing, eleven years later, we had an insight into the experience of grief caused by conflict, to the traumatic consequences of terrible events and how different people respond at different times. I could see how the deep silence of grief is made worse when bereavement arises from the active will of others. I saw how hurtful it is when efforts are made to legitimise loss and suffering in pursuit of political goals. In short, I could see that such events would have a very serious and enduring impact on those directly affected with significant personal and family health, economic and social consequences. Also, in the context of the loss arising from politically motivated violence, the efforts to grieve and heal were daily frustrated by ongoing violence and aggravated by a political discourse that was often unempathetic and brutal. I could see the problem but did not know what the solution was, other than to offer support and hope that in time people and communities would find themselves in a better place.

I also observed how, even though the events and circumstances behind grief and traumatic distress related to events and circumstances in the past, the experiences and the distress were often real and in the present. It was not surprising, therefore, that some thought they could never overcome the losses and experiences that seemed to change their lives so much. Yet, the lives of those who had experienced devastating events and circumstances and who, in time, triumphed over such experiences, revealed that there is indeed a hope of recovery.

Later, I would see that notwithstanding its benefits and desirability, peace – the cessation of violence and the development of politics – whilst it provided some succour, was not the answer for the enduring loneliness of loss, injury and trauma. Nor can it of itself make good the deep psychological rigours of other consequences of conflict, such as rejection of one's humanity, oppression, torture, the disappearance of loved ones, exile or imprisonment. In fact, for many it increased the perception of futility of past violence and, more specifically, the futility of the death of a loved one or friend, or the chronic painful injury or depression. Sometimes this gave rise to a cry to be heard. Whilst peace meant not waking to the reports on the radio of another killing or atrocity, it did not stop the nightmares. Nor could we rely upon peace alone to address the loss of faith in oneself, in others, in the world – or the loss of faith itself.

The experience of Enniskillen showed how central family, friendship, neighbourliness and community are in cradling those who suffer loss and trauma. In civil conflict however, the usual ways and means in which families, neighbourhoods and communities work are disrupted and sometimes break down. And there was always the danger of politics getting in the way of addressing the needs of individuals and families affected by violence. The voices and needs of the bereaved, injured, traumatised and of those otherwise adversely affected by violence are not readily heard when fear and mistrust dominate daily life, and when groups and actors continue to legitimise and justify violence. For those who suffer the consequences of violence, competing political commentaries upon outrages can make it seem that nothing has been learned from the spectacle of human suffering especially when events are used to reinforce political or violent positions.

Conflict also poses considerable challenges for services that support communities, and in particular those affected by violence. Through witnessing the consequences of the Enniskillen bombing it seemed to me that civic society, its institutions and services needed to find a more effective response to the needs of those who struggled with grief and trauma. For example, services could be more proactive, reaching out to the bereaved, injured and distressed rather than waiting for them to call for help. Critically, a specific understanding of the experience of loss, injury and trauma in the context of the terror and injustices of civil conflict and wider social and economic challenges, needed to shape the services being offered to, and the manner of engagement with, those affected by violence.

The structure and approach of the book

This book describes the work undertaken in Omagh against the background of the most recent period of violent conflict in Ireland, commonly referred to as 'the Troubles' a term upon which I rely to denote this period. Centrally, it draws upon the work colleagues and I undertook following the Omagh bombing.

With no time to think, colleagues and I were flung into the immediate chaos of the Omagh bombing. Shortly, however, we began to think about what needed to be done in response to this atrocity and to draw upon the experiences of Enniskillen, along with the growing knowledge about the impact of traumatic events, the intuitive and concerned responses of the community, and a changed political context. The impact of the bomb and the early responses are described in Chapters 1 and 2. Chapter 3 describes the outcome of needs-assessments undertaken following the Omagh bombing. Taking a wider and longer-term perspective and through an overview of research, Chapters 4 and 5 look in some detail at the efforts to understand the mental health and related impact of the violence associated with the Troubles in Northern Ireland over the period 1969 to 2015. Chapter 6 describes the later efforts, after the initial response in Omagh drew to a close, to build services for the benefit of the wider population, drawing upon the lessons gained in responding to the Omagh bombing. This chapter, along with Chapters, 7, 8 and 9, with reference to the work of the Northern Ireland Centre for Trauma and Transformation (NICTT), describes developments in therapy, in training and education, and in research and advocacy. Finally, Chapter 10 seeks to draw together key conclusions about the approaches that could be taken to address mental health and well-being as an essential component of a peace-building project. At the outset, a timeline is included to give a sense of the work described herein against the background of the Troubles.

The chapters that follow are written in the third person with individuals being referred to in terms of their position, role or organisation so that readers not familiar with the details of Omagh and Northern Ireland can more readily relate the text to their own circumstances. For similar reasons, some terms specific to the Troubles and in common usage in Northern Ireland have been replaced with more widely used and understood alternatives.

The work described in the following chapters relies significantly upon the idea that traumatic circumstances and experiences can disrupt – temporarily or on a more long-term basis – our mental health and well-being. In undertaking the work described, it proved helpful to think in terms of trauma-related difficulties, disorders, recovery, adjustment and growth, and to adopt a trauma-informed approach to understanding needs and to designing and providing therapeutic services. We also saw how traumatic events can unearth earlier problems. One of the concepts we relied upon for both research and therapeutic purposes was post-traumatic stress disorder (PTSD), that is, a recognisable disorder that can occur following involvement in a traumatic experience or as a result of living in traumatic and highly distressing circumstances. PTSD is one of the classified disorders described by, for example, the Diagnostic and Statistical Manual of Mental Disorders (APA, 2000). Used empathetically, and in personally and culturally relevant ways, it proved to be a useful way of thinking about the adverse psychological reactions and consequences of traumatic experiences and circumstances. It provided a way of thinking about and organising those reactions into a framework that could be widely used therapeutically to understand and address the needs of those suffering the effects of such experiences. It offered a common language across the experiences of many who suffered similar – if highly individualised – problems, and it supported the therapeutic alliance between therapeutic practitioners and those seeking help. It helped to determine the therapeutic goals of those seeking help, and to develop the skills and knowledge of practitioners. In research terms, it proved to be a very helpful lens through which to understand the scale of the impact of the Omagh bombing on the community, and later, the impact of the Troubles on the Northern Ireland population.

1

The Omagh bombing and the community's response

On the afternoon of Saturday 15 August 1998, at around 3.10 p.m., a car with a bomb on board exploded in Market Street, one of the main shopping streets in Omagh, Co. Tyrone, Northern Ireland. The explosion killed 29 adults and children, including a woman at an advanced stage of pregnancy expecting twins. Over 400 people were injured, of whom 135 suffered serious injuries; 12 children aged 0–12 years and 39 people aged 13–20 years were hospitalised (Jenkins and McKinney, 2000). Seven hospitals in Northern Ireland received casualties on the day, with two more hospitals providing specialist services in the days that followed. The bombing was the largest single incident, in terms of dead and injured, that had occurred during the civil conflict in Northern Ireland, which had commenced in 1969 (McKittrick et al., 2007). In the words of Froggatt it was 'the worst of many' examples of carnage (Froggatt, 1999: 1637). The explosion and its traumatic consequences were experienced and witnessed by thousands of people who were present at the time, or in the immediate aftermath at the scene, in the hospital nearby, and in other locations in the town.

The bombing came just four months after the Northern Ireland peace agreement, known formally as the Belfast Agreement (1998) and more informally as the Good Friday Agreement. The Agreement had been signed by the British and Irish Governments, with the support and agreement of most of the political parties in Northern Ireland, and the support of the United States of America. The bombing had been carried out by two proscribed Irish republican groups, the Real IRA (Irish Republican Army) and the Continuity IRA, which were opposed to the political settlement that had been agreed earlier in the year. Apart from the human tragedy of the bombing, the atrocity immediately gave rise to significant concerns about the stability and future of the political agreement (Dingley, 2001).

As outlined in the Introduction, two days after the bombing, the British Secretary of State with responsibility for British direct rule in Northern Ireland, Dr Marjorie Mowlam M.P. visited Omagh and met with many of those who had been directly affected, including emergency services, politicians and clergy. She also met with health and social care staff who had been involved in the immediate response to the bombing and who were already putting in place arrangements to respond to the community's needs. Dr Mowlam enquired about the immediate and longer-term implications of the bombing. She asked two important questions. The first was what the human impact would be. The second was what should be done to address the needs of people affected by the bombing. After a discussion on these fundamental questions she asked for a report and advice on how best to proceed. She was anxious that there would be no obstacles to people receiving help, and asked that strategic coordination arrangements be put in place to ensure that delays and unnecessary bureaucracy could be overcome. The report was prepared and sent to her shortly after her visit (Bolton, 1998).

Earlier in 1998, as part of the work undertaken in the development of the Belfast Agreement, Dr Mowlam had commissioned a report on the human impact of the years of civil conflict, to include recommendations on the responses required to address the identified needs. The work was undertaken by a former head of the Northern Ireland Civil Service, Sir Kenneth Bloomfield. His Report, *We Will Remember Them* (Bloomfield, 1998) was published in May 1998, some weeks after the Belfast Agreement, and three months prior to the Omagh bombing. The report described and evaluated the experiences of those affected by violence linked to the conflict, and made a number of recommendations for addressing the impact. The initiative was the first governmental comprehensive assessment of the human impact, since the most recent period of violence (the Troubles) had commenced in 1969. Another report from Northern Ireland's Department of Health and Social Services (DHSS, 1998), which was published within weeks of the Belfast Agreement had made further recommendations focusing on some health and social care issues. In the wake of the Omagh bombing, these reports and their recommendations created new possibilities and expectations as to how the impact of the bombing could and would be addressed.

The initial responses to the bombing

Within minutes of the bombing, the local hospital in Omagh, The Tyrone County Hospital, which was located less than a kilometre away from the scene, began to receive casualties. The small accident and emergency facility was quickly overwhelmed and other areas of the hospital were put into service to receive and treat casualties. The ambulance service and local people brought casualties to hospital in cars, taxis and commandeered buses. Soon after, helicopters from the nearby army base began to transfer seriously ill casualties to the regional trauma centres in Derry/Londonderry and Belfast, and the overflow of less seriously injured to the sub-regional hospitals in Enniskillen and Dungannon. Local general and military medical practitioners also provided immediate treatment. Staff from the hospital who were on leave went to the hospital after a public appeal for help that was broadcast on radio and television. Medical, nursing and various health and social care practitioners from other parts of Northern Ireland and the Republic of Ireland came to Omagh to assist. Practitioners from other places who were in or close to Omagh on the day also offered their help.

Alongside the care and treatment of the casualties, a large number of people from the local community, who were concerned for relatives and friends, began to gather at the hospital seeking information. Community-based health and social care staff and staff from local not-for-profit organisations, working with the hospital staff, quickly set up arrangements to assist those who were seeking information about relatives. The demands were such that it was decided to move the missing relative enquiry service off the hospital site to the nearby Omagh District Council leisure centre, at the invitation of the Council's chief executive. This was a very suitable facility, providing large spaces for people to gather, private areas, toilets, telephones and a restaurant, and was very accessible to the hospital and other key facilities in the town, such as the temporary mortuary at the local Army barracks. The decision also had the effect of diverting many hundreds of people from the hospital to an alternative location, providing more space at the hospital for the care and treatment of the casualties, and space and privacy for their families. Also, the focus of the media at this stage was on the hospital. This meant that the response team at the leisure centre was able, at least in the early hours, to carry out a sensitive and complex task with bereaved families without a large media presence.

Within hours, and continuing over the following thirty-six hours, the leisure centre became the focal point for coordinating details about the location and movements of people who were reported missing and those who had been transferred to the regional hospitals. Later in the evening on the day of the bombing, details of those who were missing and unaccounted for were coordinated by police and health and social care staff with information about those who had been killed. Preliminary information about the possible death of loved ones was shared with families, whilst further information was being sought. The rupture of a major telephone cable in the explosion, along with the heavy traffic on both landlines and mobile phone systems, meant that there were great difficulties in communications. Fortunately one telephone line from the leisure centre remained operational throughout and this was restricted to urgent telephone calls with, for example, the nearby hospital, the police casualty bureau in Belfast, and regional hospitals.

Towards midnight, family representatives of those who were missing and believed to be dead, police, staff from the leisure centre, local clergy and the health and social care team assembled in a more private room to be briefed on the arrangements that would follow to undertake identification of the dead. The senior manager with the Sperrin Lakeland Health and Social Care Trust (the local public health services provider) and the senior police officer, who were coordinating the efforts to locate the missing and identify those who had been killed, briefed the gathering. The proposals on how identifications would be undertaken were outlined. It was going to take a long time and families were offered assistance to go home if they wished to change clothes or to allow another family member to take their place at the leisure centre. This solemn and sad gathering concluded with a short address by the chief executive of Omagh Council, and with prayers by two Christian church leaders, the Catholic Bishop of Derry and the President of the Methodist Church in Ireland.

Throughout the night, family-by-family, relatives were brought to the temporary mortuary at the army barracks by the police, supported by each family's choice of clergy, friends and other relatives, or health and social care staff, to undertake the identifications. The arrangements for those who had died and for their identification were very sensitively put in place by the army with advice from Omagh's most senior police officer and the Sperrin Lakeland's community services director. A sports pavilion was made available as an anteroom, where tea and coffee were provided, and where families could gather and be briefed by the police on what would take place. Next door was the viewing room, which had been carefully prepared in a short time with flowers and appropriate furniture to be as respectful and supportive as possible. Depending on the religious denomination of the family, religious artefacts were assembled in the room for each identification. Some families had more than one person to identify. After the formalities of identification were over and families had spent some time with their deceased relative, they withdrew to the anteroom, where they were given time to compose themselves and where any questions they had could be addressed, before returning to the leisure centre. These arrangements also overcame the added difficulty of bringing identifying relatives into a mortuary where there were deceased persons, other than their family members. Considering there were, at that point, twenty-eight deaths, this took all of Saturday night and well into Sunday. It was a very difficult period for the families, who were greatly distressed. Many of those who had died, or their families, were known personally to staff from the police, the leisure centre, the clergy and the health and social care team, which included staff from not-for-profit agencies. The loss of so many, and the evident distress of their families, was deeply felt by all. Who could have imagined that a day could end like this?

The human impact

By the following afternoon the number of deaths was confirmed at twenty-eight, including the woman carrying twins. It became and remained important for the community to remember the twins in the deadly toll of the bombing. At that point, one person was unaccounted for but was subsequently confirmed to have been elsewhere at the time of the bombing. Another man was to die from his injuries three weeks later. Two days after the bombing a man died in a collision between his car and an ambulance transferring patients between hospitals. He and his family were subsequently remembered as an indirect casualty and bereaved family of the bombing.

Of the over 400 who had been injured, 135 were very seriously injured, with severe burns, severe soft tissue injuries or traumatic amputations. It was also clear that thousands of people had been exposed in one way or another to the experience of the bomb explosion or its immediate traumatic consequences. This included those who were in Market Street, where the bomb had exploded, and those who had felt the explosion from nearby shops, car parks or other streets, many of whom went to Market Street in search of relatives or to offer assistance. The scene immediately after the explosion was profoundly traumatic. Others who were at a greater distance or in their homes and who heard the explosion also came in search of relatives whom they believed might be in the town shopping or working. Soon after, the emergency services began to arrive and they too were faced with a scene of devastation and seriously injured adults and children. Then, in the first hour or so, many who gathered at the hospital witnessed scenes of the seriously injured being brought in ambulances or in improvised and commandeered vehicles to the accident and emergency department. They witnessed great distress amongst those who were seeking relatives or who had otherwise been caught up in the tragedy. The urgency and scale of the situation meant that many civilians witnessed scenes that would normally only be seen by those directly involved, and by emergency service personnel in the most extreme situations. Later, similar scenes played themselves out in the leisure centre and the temporary mortuary, and in many homes across the town, in nearby villages and the countryside. Additonally, the impact of the bomb was felt beyond Omagh, in Buncrana in Co. Donegal, and Madrid, Spain, from where some of those killed and injured came. This was a deeply felt community tragedy for adults and children and their families and friends from the Omagh district, from both the nationalist and unionist traditions, with wider and international repercussions.

How the longer-term response took shape

It was clear within hours that the bombing posed a serious mental health risk for the bereaved, the injured, families, witnesses, rescuers, networks of friends and colleagues, school and faith communities, and those who had been involved in the care, treatment and support of casualties and the bereaved. Within hours, work began on putting together a strategy for addressing the mental health impacts. This would involve a range of interventions and responses, which are discussed in more detail below.

Whilst at one level the impact was understood, there was a need to communicate the impact and risks in a way that would stimulate and support urgent and appropriate policy and service responses. Concerns were expressed by the public,

Table 1: Framework for considering the impact of community tragedies

Less negative impact	←——————→	More negative impact
Expected		Unexpected
Contained		Extensive
Low horror		Intense horror
Few losses		Multiple loss
No displacement		Extensive displacement
No disruption		Extensive disruption
Control maintained		High loss of control
Minimal uncertainty		Sustained uncertainty
A shared and common view		Conflicting understanding
Accidental or natural		Inflicted/human cause

community organisations, family doctors services and mental health services about the psychological and mental health risks that would follow the bombing. However, it was not until the major studies discussed in Chapter 3 were undertaken that it was possible to provide robust estimates of the psychological impact of the bombing. In the meantime, politicians, service commissioners and civil servants wanted some assessment of the impact and a way of expressing this. There was a parallel need to provide a sense of hope and expectation of recovery for the community, as many in positions of leadership were concerned at the community, political and service implications. On sensing the scale of the human devastation caused by the bombing, one senior politician expressed deep concern as to how a community could possibly ever recover from such a blow and was at a loss to know what might be done politically to address the personal and communal consequences.

To convey where the bombing registered as a community tragedy, reference was made to a framework developed some years earlier to reflect upon the impact of the Enniskillen bombing of 1987 (Table 1). The framework provided a short series of questions that could be posed about community tragedies and their psychological and social implications, upon which decisions and actions could be based (Bolton, 1999: 203).

Using the framework to assess the impact of the bombing, a picture emerged of a significantly toxic psychological event in the life of the Omagh community, with potential risks for the psychological well-being of individuals, and associated social and economic implications. The bombing:

- was unexpected;
- was intensely horrific;
- led to multiple losses and casualties;
- caused extensive disruption (both in community and political terms);

- led to significant loss of community control and stability, or was in serious danger of doing so;
- produced profound political and personal uncertainty;
- arose out of circumstances with origins that are a profound matter of ideological and political dispute;
- was an act of aggression i.e. had a human cause.

The framework provided a systematic basis upon which judgments could be made about the likely consequences of the bombing and thereby provided decision makers with a rationale for action. It was used to support the explanation as to what the impact of the bombing could be and to make the case for investment in appropriate responses. The analysis derived from the framework was included in a number of documents and presentations on the impact of the bombing, and formed part of the case for developing services and seeking funding. Generally, funders, agencies with responsibilities and people in positions of authority welcomed it as a basis for understanding the tragedy and its consequences, and as a basis for planning and service development.

The early response – the development of mental health services

On the Monday morning after the explosion, a multiagency centre for those who were affected by the bombing was opened. This would address practical needs (housing, welfare benefits, loss of employment), disability related and welfare needs, and the emotional and psychological needs of the local population. An available building was opened for this purpose on the main street of the town. Links began to be established between local publicly provided health and social care services and not-for-profit services such as Victim Support (a regional non-governmental organisation which was already providing services in the Omagh District), The Samaritans (a largely telephone based helpline for people experiencing psychological distress) and the Tara Centre, a local community focused counselling and personal development organisation. Local family doctor and mental health services started to receive requests for assistance from those with minor injuries and with acute psychological distress. It was later estimated that over the course of the four weeks following the bombing, family doctors had 2,500 additional contacts, over and above their baseline work, as a result of the bombing. Together, in the first month, the local not-for-profit organisations and the family doctor services responded to a significant demand from the local population, principally for support in relation to psychological difficulties.

Meanwhile, the local public health and social care provider, The Sperrin Lakeland Health and Social Care Trust, began to implement its emergency plans. This included establishing what became the Omagh Community Trauma and Recovery Team. The origins, aims and work of the Team are discussed in more detail in Chapter 2. The Trust had a duty, required by Northern Ireland's health department (the DHSS), as part of the emergency planning response to any major incident, to put in place a longer-term psychological support service. The Trust was the provider of both local hospital services (including those at the Tyrone County Hospital that had responded initially on the day of the explosion) and community services such as disability, mental health and family and child care services. It was responsible for the delivery of primary care services and for liaison and coordination with local family doctor services. (The Trust was one of Northern Ireland's public integrated health and social care service providers.) There was also a well-established pattern of liaison and cooperation with not-for-profit and private service providers operating in the area and with local community groups and partnerships and with local private sector providers of social care. In addition, because of the bombing, new connections were made or amplified with, for example, the education system through the local education headquarters in Omagh, senior managers of local schools, and local church and faith community leaders. This comprehensive network of responsibilities, plus established and new relationships, meant that the Trust, acting under its duty to provide long-term psychological care, had a key role to play.

Public, political and media expectations

As a result of the highly charged political context of the tragedy, additional expectations became apparent, with politicians and community leaders being concerned that services should be provided for those affected by the bombing. The Victims Commissioner's Report (Bloomfield, 1998) had created a framework and expectations for the response to be provided. As a result, those responsible for policy in relation to those affected by the conflict (i.e. politicians and civil servants) and those affected by the tragedy had expectations on what form the response to the bombing should take.

The need to articulate the nature of the impact and the response was pressing, in view of the enquiries the Trust was receiving from the British Government's Northern Ireland Office, regional and local political parties and representatives, Northern Ireland's health department and media. Views were also being expressed and questions raised by authorities in the Republic of Ireland given the impact of the bombing on the Buncrana community in north Donegal, and from the Spanish embassies in Dublin and London. In the first week after the bombing senior managers with the Trust dealt with numerous political and media enquiries on these matters. The problem facing the Trust's senior managers was that, whilst they knew that the bombing was having – and would have – serious psychological consequences, it was not clear what the nature and scale of this impact would be. Likewise, in the context of a conventional mental health service and an under-developed trauma-focused service and capability, it was not clear what form the response should or could take. Nevertheless, drawing upon the experiences of some of the senior managers and practitioners in responding to other tragedies, chiefly those associated with the Troubles, plans were developed and put in place. Key to working through this complexity was the leadership of the Trust's chief executive. He assimilated the evidence coming from within the Trust and from the wider community, including its politicians, and acting with the support of the Trust's chairman and board, quickly authorised the actions required to move things forward and put in place appropriate services.

Coordinating and managing the response

To coordinate the health and social care response to the bombing, three main structures were put in place in line with the Trust's emergency plans. First was an interagency committee, which comprised senior representatives of all the public bodies with relevant responsibilities, including the local District Council, the police, the housing authority and the education services. Senior managers and practitioners from within the Sperrin Lakeland Trust represented its key service departments, including its disability and mental health services. Senior officials from the Trust's health and social care services commissioning agency, the Western Health and Social Services Board, were included, as well as civil servants from the Victims Liaison Unit, which had been established by the Northern Ireland Office to take forward the recommendations of the Victims Commissioner's Report (also referred to as the Bloomfield Report) (Bloomfield, 1998). Faith communities and not-for-profit service providers were also represented. This committee was chaired by the chief executive of the Trust and met frequently in the early weeks and months after the bombing.

The two other structures, focusing chiefly on the psychological and health related needs of the population and associated services, were a not-for-profit services forum and an internal Sperrin Lakeland Trust services committee. The not-for-profit services forum brought together the trust and providers from the not-for-profit sector that were providing support, counselling and other related services, including those providing practical care such as the British Red Cross and the Knights of Malta organisations. The experience of the forum highlighted the benefits of having clear arrangements and agreements in place so that each agency and sector could play its part, acting upon its strengths in the wake of a major community tragedy. It was also an important context for exchanging information on events and other developments and proved to be a useful mechanism for coordinating responses to the bombing. In the first year it coordinated central funding support for not-for-profit sector organisations. Whilst it was not the place to share information about individuals, due to some organisational difficulties the forum was unable to pool general information about identified needs and the use and impact of services. As a consequence it was not possible to establish an overview of the needs identified and the services addressed by the not-for-profit sector in the first year.

The internal committee within the Sperrin Lakeland Trust, which coordinated the response of its hospital and community services, drew together these services and included disability, home and primary care, mental health and rehabilitation services. This was particularly helpful in ensuring that family support, home care and disability services were acting to support the therapeutic work of the Omagh Community Trauma and Recovery Team (discussed further in Chapter 2), and that liaison arrangements between the Team and the mental health services were in place. There remained a challenge of balancing the very significant and sudden demands for services arising from the bombing and maintaining services to other patients and clients. Given the community context of the tragedy, staff whose chief role was to maintain existing services would from time to time find, on visiting a home in the community for example, that the family had been seriously affected. Also, some people with long-term mental health problems found their conditions worsened as a consequence of the bombing with consequences for them and their families.

These groups met weekly in the early months after the bombing, with reduced frequency thereafter, and were wound up after the first anniversary when systems had become well established. Both groups and the Omagh Community Trauma and Recovery Team were coordinated by the Trust's director of community care. Besides their specific functions, these structures provided opportunities for exploratory conversations amongst key actors in the response to the bombing, helped to shape further developments, afforded opportunities for explanations to be provided about needs or service requirements etc., and addressed matters that had given rise to confusion, speculation and misunderstandings.

Over-arching these arrangements was the role of the Sperrin Lakeland Trust's senior management team and its board of executive and non-executive directors. In the first week after the bombing, the management team, chaired by the chief executive, met every morning at 8.00 a.m. and in the evening – sometimes with other meetings during the working day. The complex impact of the bombing, coupled with the Trust's broad range of emergency, hospital and community responsibilities, gave rise to a very intense period of work, which required much senior managerial attention over the following months, continuing until after the first anniversary. To this was added the very large number of offers of help and of condolences, the large number of media enquiries and the liaison with regional hospitals, senior civil servants and politicians, all of which added another layer of complexity. This aspect was specifically coordinated and managed by one of the Trust's directors.

Moving to address the mental health impacts

In the period immediately after the bombing, the focus was on the injured and their need for hospital and rehabilitation services. There was also the need to connect patients, some of whom were very seriously ill, with more specialist services – which often meant movement from the local hospitals in Omagh and Enniskillen to the more specialist centres in Derry/Londonderry and greater Belfast. Meanwhile the Omagh hospital was endeavouring to resume normal services, as many planned hospital admissions and out-patient clinics had been cancelled following the explosion so the full resources of the hospital could be deployed in response to the bombing. Shortly, the focus began to shift to the needs of those who required rehabilitation and to the needs of those with mental health needs, of which there was growing awareness.

Some weeks following the bombing, and in an effort to find out more about the wider community's views, needs and ideas on how best to respond, an invitation was extended by the Sperrin Lakeland Trust to community leaders, service providers and others who were interested in joining in a conversation. This took the form of a day-long meeting held in the leisure centre which had played a key role in the immediate aftermath of the bombing. All who attended were invited to contribute their thoughts on a range of issues and questions that had been determined and refined at the start of the meeting. This gathering provided an opportunity to hear more detailed and nuanced insights into the impact of the bombing, to hear things that were encouraging, and about other previously unnoticed concerns. It also helped create a sense of common purpose and facilitated contact amongst people occupying key roles who otherwise might not have had any or much previous personal contact. The meeting produced a number of observations and recommendations, a summary of which was distributed to all who attended and to other agencies and individuals in the community.

Occupational health services and other responses

The bombing had a major impact on business owners and employees of shops and businesses working in the locality of the bombing. Many of those who died or were injured were well known as colleagues, customers and friends of the local shops and businesses, and the sense of loss and shock was very much felt by this part of the community. Staff of the emergency and other services who were called upon to respond to the bombing were also affected by their experiences, with many reporting short-term intense distress, and some developing longer-term emotional and psychological difficulties. Major public bodies had various arrangements for staff care and support. Local businesses generally used local health services, and some franchise and chain stores had access to corporate staff care support arrangements.

In the Sperrin Lakeland Trust, staff care arrangements were a principal matter of concern for its occupational health and staff support services. The Trust's occupational health consultant took the view that the bombing gave rise to two main risks for staff, one being the high level of exposure to body tissues and fluids with associated risks, the other being the high level of exposure to traumatic experiences. Strategies were put in place by the occupational health department to address both these concerns. In relation to the psychological risks, the Sperrin Lakeland Trust's staff support arrangements were mobilised. This involved internal staff support services and external independent staff care services. Also, some trades unions and professional bodies offered support to their members. Hospital chaplains and other faith leaders contributed through informal staff focused ceremonies aimed at acknowledging what had happened and the role staff had played in the response. Senior managers, executive and non-executive directors of the Sperrin Lakeland Trust visited the hospital and other facilities involved in the response, offering support to staff, patients and others involved or otherwise affected by the tragedy. Staff teams supported each other, mindful, for example, of the needs of those who would be on their own whilst off duty. Also, many staff and their families had been affected directly by the bombing, with many others feeling deeply the impact of a community tragedy because of the consequences for colleagues, neighbours and friends. Later, key public figures and politicians visited the hospital and other service locations to meet patients and families, and to acknowledge and express appreciation for the response of local services to the bombing. This complex response within the health and social care services, repeated across the community and its institutions, at times carefully planned, at other points very spontaneous, contributed much to the community efforts to deal with a shared and very distressing experience.

Responding to the concerns of the wider community

The bombing was both a major human tragedy and a political and community relations crisis. Within hours, the media were carrying public condemnations of the attack, chiefly from political leaders and figures, and from other governments. Over the following weeks, senior public figures and political leaders visited Omagh, including the British Prime Minister, Tony Blair; the Irish Taoiseach, Bertie Ahern; Prince Charles from the British royal family; the President of Ireland, Mary McAleese; and the President of the United States of America, Bill Clinton, who included Omagh in a last minute change of plan to a scheduled visit to Ireland. These visits were major events in themselves, requiring high levels of interagency planning and giving rise to major security considerations, with considerable implications for the Omagh Council, the police service and other public bodies.

In the hours and days following the bombing, flowers began to be laid at key locations in Omagh, chiefly at the site of the bombing and nearby, and at the Tyrone County Hospital where the front lawn would soon be covered in flowers. At times lorry loads of floral tributes were arriving in the town, particularly from the Republic of Ireland where there was a very widespread desire to stand alongside those who had been affected by the bombing, which had been carried out in pursuance of the republican aim of achieving a united Ireland. In time, the large quantity of flowers gave rise to a major problem – how to respectfully dispose of tons of flowers, which were rapidly becoming an environmental and public health risk? How this matter was addressed is discussed further below.

As already noted, many varying offers of help were made, from many different sources. This included offers of holidays, clothing, gifts of various kinds, offers of meeting others affected by similar tragedies and trauma counselling or therapies. Also, very soon, gifts of money were arriving in Omagh and the District Council had to rapidly put in place mechanisms to receive and eventually disburse funds that were offered in support of those who had been bereaved, injured and psychologically traumatised. To this end, the Omagh Fund was established. Guided by responses to previous tragedies, the legal arrangements were put in place to authorise this not-for-profit body of trustees to receive and disburse funds. By the time the Fund closed in 2002, over £6 million had been received and distributed. Once the Fund was established, even more offers of support were received, along with further offers to raise funds. This led to events such as football matches in Omagh between the local football club and Manchester United, Chelsea and Liverpool clubs, and the production of music albums – the proceeds of which contributed to the Fund. The Fund's chairman and trustees were committed to ensuring that those in need of assistance received it as quickly as possible. Initial payments were made to the families of the bereaved and seriously injured within weeks, with more payments made thereafter based on assessments of the impact of the bombing and of need. For a time, some funds were retained so that, in the event of advances in technology or medicine, or in the event of changing circumstances, there was the prospect of the Fund assisting with interventions that would help those who were injured to further overcome any limitations they had experienced as a result of the bombing. The chairman and trustees of the Fund were also concerned that they should be in a position to bring assistance to those who had suffered psychological problems, recognising in particular that some with such problems would only emerge much later, and that many who were so affected would need access to specialist trauma-focused therapeutic services. This advocacy on behalf of those suffering psychological problems significantly influenced the work of the original Omagh Team and later the NICTT, and the Fund provided financial support to several local organisations so that therapeutic services were available to people affected by the bombing.

Ceremonial and arts-based responses to the bombing

In Northern Ireland Christian churches still play a very important role in the lives of many, particularly in relation to moments of crisis and for rites of passage relating to birth, marriage and death. Working with other faiths, the Omagh Churches' Forum played a significant part in commenting on the tragedy and its impact and in assisting the community in marking it in different ways, chiefly through the funerals in the days after the bombing and through major acts of public worship. The funerals of those who had died were themselves major community events, with large numbers attending, especially those in the greater Omagh area and Buncrana in Co. Donegal. While the larger community and national responses were unfolding, in each of the church and other faith communities affected by the bombing, family funerals were being arranged. This, along with the pastoral needs of those who had been injured, placed considerable demands upon families, clergy, other faith leaders and congregations.

One out of many formal and informal community events is worthy of particular note. A week after the bombing, tens of thousands of people stood along Omagh's main street facing up towards the courthouse from where the ceremony was led. The event was organised to acknowledge what had happened, to give thanks for the lives of those who had been lost, to remember the injured and bereaved and to acknowledge the unknown but immense number of acts of human kindness that had been unleashed by the tragedy. The ceremony had been quickly arranged and its liturgy prepared to include clergy representing many of the Christian denominations and representatives of the public services and volunteer agencies that had responded to the bombing. The event was televised live in Northern Ireland and in other countries, including the Republic of Ireland and Britain. Whilst there were many words, in some senses both those who took part and those who were present were in a place which words could not easily reach. Yet the familiar passages from the Bible and the recognisable and expected intentions of the prayers and hymns were a point of connection, a source of comfort and consolation. The sheer scale of the gathering was itself totemic and there was a real sense in which those gathered wanted to be there, for themselves, for each other and for the community, as an act of solidarity and an act of protest. The most striking moment of the ceremony was when local singer, Juliet Turner, sang Julie Miller's song 'Broken Things' (Miller, 1993). The song and the performance transfixed those who were there, as they seemed to express so much of what, at that point, had not yet been expressed. This ceremony, which brought people together with its familiar and unfamiliar words and music, its moments of silence, and the reciting of the names of those who had died, offered a profoundly moving and helpful avenue, through which those who had gathered and the communities they represented could begin to get to grips with this overwhelming tragedy.

Another significant response was the Petals of Hope project. Artist Carole Kane, responding to public discussions about how the enormous amounts of floral tributes should be respectfully disposed of, suggested a way in which this sensitive task could be undertaken. She proposed a series of workshops involving local volunteers who together created a series of collages with handmade paper manufactured and decorated with dried flowers and leaves from the floral tributes. One piece was made for each of those who had died, including a piece for the unborn twins, and three larger pieces representing each of the three communities affected by the tragedy, Buncrana in Co. Donegal, Madrid in Spain and Omagh. The collection formed part of an exhibition 'Petals of Hope – Rays of Light' which was exhibited in Omagh, Dublin, Belfast and Buncrana in the spring and early summer of 1999 and is also the subject of a publication (Kane, 1999).

The role of the media

The bombing and its consequences inevitably resulted in intense local, national and international media attention. The news-worthiness of the tragedy was evident given its scale and political significance, following as it did after the Belfast Agreement, and its international dimensions. In an age of 24-hour news coverage it was inevitable that there would be immense media interest. The author recalls his experience in 1987 following the Enniskillen Remembrance Sunday bombing when there were two prototype satellite television vehicles in the town in the first week or so following that tragedy. In Omagh, eleven years later, on one day shortly after the bombing, there were 40 such vehicles in the designated media park.

Whilst the news coverage did not explicitly have therapeutic aims, there was considerable sensitivity on the part of media in the first year after the bombing. Of particular note was the reporting by the local weekly newspapers in Omagh, the *Ulster Herald* and the *Tyrone Constitution*, both of which covered the bombing and what followed in considerable detail. Over the months and years that followed, the sensitive coverage by the two newspapers provided informed opportunities for a whole range of experiences and events to be reported upon, and provided valuable information for the public. On the occasion of the commemoration that took place a week after the bombing, when tens of thousands gathered not far from where the bomb had exploded, a prayer was said, giving thanks for the role of the media, 'for telling our story to the world' (Mullan and Herron et al., 1998). There was much appreciation locally that the story of the bombing and its impact had been told comprehensively, and for the acknowledgement it brought to the Omagh community. Some of the coverage portrayed the deep personal, family and community tragedy that had been experienced. The media's interest facilitated a conversation and the sharing of narratives about the bombing.

Conversely, for some, media coverage was a source of distress, particularly in relation to distressing accounts of events and later, when controversies arose about the political, security and policing aspects of the run-up to and response to the bombing. Likewise, video footage of the bombing was often used by television programmes for illustration purposes, which were sometimes only indirectly related to the subject of the Omagh bombing itself. At times, those caught up in the tragedy felt emotionally ambushed by such use of films and images, as they had not had time to anticipate and prepare for particular occasions of their usage. In some cases people chose not to watch television for periods of time when they felt particularly vulnerable.

Media agencies and reporters sought to examine and clarify what people's needs were and also what services would be available to meet those needs. Within days not-for-profit and publicly provided health and social care services were being asked about what they were doing in response to the bombing and what would be available to the public. As noted earlier, in the first week after the bombing, there was an expectation in political circles, which was picked up by some media sources, that counselling would be readily and immediately available. This expectation created a number of problems which staff from the Sperrin Lakeland Trust sought to rebalance. First, broadly speaking, the attention of the community, even of those who were experiencing emotional and psychological problems, was on those who had died and on their funerals, which took place over the course of the first seven days. Second, it was considered that counselling (i.e. therapy services) would be required in due course by a proportion of adults and children in the wider community who would go on to suffer on-going and serious psychological and mental health difficulties. However, so soon after the tragedy, counselling would not be generally an appropriate response. Within days of the tragedy the focus should be on social support, minimising isolation, promoting constructive collective and personal responses and creating an expectation of recovery from short-term distress – whilst encouraging people to seek help if problems persisted or worsened. Meanwhile, work commenced on developing services to provide support in the short term, principally through the family doctor and primary care services and a number of not-for-profit sector organisations, and on developing medium- and longer-term therapeutic services. Also, in the first few weeks the on-going support of bereaved families through the police family liaison services and other publicly provided and not-for-profit agencies continued, as did the support of those who were injured, through the surgical, medical, primary care and rehabilitatory, disability and family services. Through responding to questions from the media on such matters, and by reports in local newspapers, key messages were conveyed on what services were available or might be developed. The local newspapers, in particular, played a key role over the first few years after the bombing, taking an interest in the progress of services, and the demands on those services. They were also willing to carry information-based reports on needs and services, particularly at key times such as when the needs-assessments described in Chapter 3 were undertaken, when the early anniversaries were happening and at the time of the inquests into the deaths arising from the bombing. One of the areas assessed in the Omagh Adult Community Study was the role of the media, which is discussed further in Chapter 3.

Conclusions

This chapter has sought to set the scene for what follows, and to describe some of the key responses by the Omagh community and its agencies to the crisis of the bombing and its anticipated long-term implications. The responses to the bombing were a feature of the moment, of the personal and community tragedy it represented and the political crisis it gave rise to. The responses were often spontaneous, intuitive and creative, with the unexpected and surprising making their contribution. The role of disaster planning played its part chiefly in ensuring that key people had the authority to act and the resources to deploy, and that there were systems in place to coordinate the responses of agencies and the community. Regarding mental health risks, the responses were influenced by knowledge about loss, trauma and the experiences of other tragedies in the life of a community and its people. The bombing gave rise to a tragedy the like of which had been never been experienced before in Omagh. In a sectarian context, the community could have fragmented and its institutions could have been immobilised or at odds. Key to the response of the greater Omagh community was the cohesiveness of its people, plus the contribution and stabilising role of its church and faith communities, and the work of its education services and local school communities, the District Council, community and not-for-profit organisations, and local health and social services – which, when faced with a tragedy that could have led to even more tragedies, found another way to respond to the shared human calamity of a summer's day.

2

The Omagh Community Trauma and Recovery Team

Within hours of the bombing, as its scale and impact and the levels of exposure to loss and trauma became apparent, it was clear to those involved in delivering the public welfare and psychological responses to the bombing that some longer-term service would be needed. The need for a focal point for the public that would provide pathways to relevant services was considered to be a priority for the local community. What became the Omagh Community Trauma and Recovery Team was established by the Sperrin Lakeland Trust within 48 hours of the bombing. It was so named to reflect the reality of the tragedy that had occurred. Its name sought to convey the hope and expectation that, in so far as was possible, some kind of recovery would be experienced by the community, mindful that after such events, life for many is never the same again. Those thoughts became important guiding principles and orientations in the face of what was felt by many, including local people and political leaders, to be an overwhelming and devastating event from which recovery could barely be conceived.

Northern Ireland had a significant and developing publicly provided mental health service that served the general and more specialist needs of the population. Notwithstanding the availability of such services in the Omagh area, it was concluded by the Sperrin Lakeland Trust that the scale and type of demand from the public in the wake of the bombing would require additional measures. Key to the development of the Team and its services was a commitment by the Trust at both senior managerial and senior practitioner levels to learn as much as possible about what the practical and psychological needs of the local community were as a result of the bombing, for the benefit of those affected by the tragedy. This included gathering data about needs and the effectiveness of services. It was hoped that these aims would be adopted by the wider public services and agencies in the not-for-profit sector. These ambitions were driven by the hope that the Omagh bombing would be the last atrocity of the recent conflict in Northern Ireland – and that this placed upon those involved in developing and delivering therapeutic services the responsibility of learning as much as possible. A further intention was that the learning from the work after the bombing would be shared widely across Northern Ireland to support service developments for others affected by the Troubles.

The opportunity to take this approach was advanced by both the considerable political interest in the tragedy and support for actions to address the needs arising from it. The hope and possibilities were also enhanced by developments in recent years in trauma research and diagnostics, which opened up new possibilities. In the early years of the Troubles much less was known about the effects of traumatic experiences and about trauma disorders. By the time of the Omagh bombing, a body of evidence was beginning to form which was pointing to a significant impact from the years of violence (see Chapters 4 and 5). The low level of evidence of the impact of loss and trauma linked to the violence from the early years of the Troubles, along with the absence of early and on-going population-wide studies into the impact, undoubtedly contributed to poor progress on policy and services. At service and practice levels, no population-wide and systematic Troubles-focused response in terms of assessment of need, referral and the provision of therapeutic interventions, was in place.

The processes that led to the Belfast Agreement included the publication of the first Victims Commissioner's Report (Bloomfield, 1998) and a report from Northern Ireland's health department (DHSS, 1998), both published just weeks after the Agreement. These signalled that those who had been bereaved, injured or suffered adverse mental health consequences as a result of the Troubles had needs relating to acknowledgement, loss and trauma. The reports also recognised the need for responses to the problems that had arisen as a consequence. In the light of later research and developments in practice, the understanding of the nature of those needs and the service requirements were limited. However, given these were two publicly sponsored reports – one with high political status, the other with a central health policy advice focus – they provided a basis for further research and development in policy and services. As far as the Omagh bombing was concerned, the reports provided the most recent policy framework. As noted earlier, they also generated expectations on the part of those affected by the tragedy, the media, politicians and strategic service managers, as to what the response to the bombing should be.

Establishing the Omagh Community Trauma and Recovery Team

Setting up, urgently, a new service at a moment of crisis was itself a challenge, although that sense of crisis and flux created a context for the unthinkable and the extraordinary. Once the decision was taken by the local public health and social care services provider, the Sperrin Lakeland Trust, to establish a trauma team to respond to the bombing, an experienced social work manager – with, amongst other things, a background in mental health, psychotherapy and disability services – was appointed as team leader. The Team itself was made up of health and social care practitioners drawn chiefly from the Trust's own services and initially was comprised of social workers, psychiatrists, psychologists, mental health nurses, an occupational therapist, an art therapist and a family therapist. Importantly, the Team had links directly into all the relevant services within the Trust, including disability, rehabilitation, family and childcare, mental health services, primary, community, hospital and home-care services. Links were also formed with schools and education services, local churches and faith communities, not-for-profit services and community organisations. After a short period based at the multiagency centre described in Chapter 1, the Team moved to its longer-term location close to, but importantly not at, the location of the bombing. It remained there for the most of the three-and-a-half years it served the community.

The profile of the Team's practitioners changed as time went on. After the first year, the focus shifted from being broadly psycho-socially based to the provision of more specialist trauma-focused therapy for individuals suffering trauma-related disorders. Staff with cognitive behavioural therapy (CBT) experience and qualifications became more involved in its therapeutic work, including an experienced psychiatrist with extensive qualifications and experience in CBT, who became the coordinator and clinical lead and supervisor of this aspect of the Team's work. Many of the staff came from the Trust's mental health teams, which assisted with the liaison and linkages to the work being undertaken by the wider mental health services.

The key functions of the Team were described in the strategy and implementation arrangements document prepared for the government. They were to:

- symbolically represent the Sperrin Lakeland Trust's response to the bombing;
- act as the spearhead for the Trust's services;
- act as an easy point of access for the community to the full range of Trust services;
- provide initial responses including assessment and services for people affected by the bombing;
- proactively and appropriately refer to the Trust's conventional services;
- coordinate the Trust's response with that of the not-for-profit sector;
- stimulate appropriate initiatives in response to the bombing to address health and social care needs;
- collate information to inform decision making and to assist research and audit;
- appropriately bring to an end the Trust's response in an agreed manner and time scale. (Bolton, 1998: 14)

In the early days, the Team focused on those seeking help for acute stress and trauma reactions to their experiences, and on working alongside the police family liaison service to support bereaved families. The Team liaised extensively with local services and organisations and provided guidance, training and briefings for local community groups and services, businesses and employers, and church groups on how people might be affected by their experience, how best they might be supported, and where they could be referred to for additional help. These briefings provided an invaluable opportunity to hear directly about how the bombing was affecting individuals, families and the wider community, about how this was changing over time, and what people's desires were in terms of public and ceremonial responses. They were an opportunity to hear about what kind of services people wanted or were likely to need, and to have conversations about the grief-related and psychological needs of those who had experienced the bombing and its consequences.

The series of meetings and contacts included an intense period of work with the management boards and staff of local schools under the guidance and imprimatur of the chief executive and senior managers of the local education authority. Through this, teachers were assisted in responding to the needs of children and young people, some of whom were bereaved by the deaths of family members or friends, who had friends or family who were injured, or in some cases who were injured themselves. The schools and the education service were also making a very significant contribution to addressing the impact of the bombing, with some very inspirational things being undertaken in schools aimed at supporting children, and by the education authority's educational welfare and educational psychology departments and staff. Ceremonial and arts-based initiatives exemplified the distinctive responses by the schools, aided in some places by external support that had been secured by the education authority (Capewell and Pittman, 1998; Pittman, 2000).

The wider community response

The team's focus on the community and personal health consequences of the bombing formed part of a raft of responses by key sectors in the Omagh community. This included the Christian churches and other faith communities, which were coordinated largely by the local Churches' Forum. The Forum had already been in place prior to the bombing and this created a valuable set of established relationships across denominations. This was important given the way in which the religious structures in Northern Ireland mark the sectarian and community divisions and fault lines. The work of the churches formed a key part of the response and leadership, providing, for example, pastoral support for families and congregations, and valuable reflections on the personal and collective tragedy, as well as modelling how the community and its various organisations and institutions might respond. The churches, other faith communities and the Forum were central to the organisation of key liturgical and ceremonial responses. This work was made visible by the joint efforts of two local clergy, a Presbyterian minister and a Catholic priest, one from each of the two main Christian traditions in Northern Ireland. They, working with colleagues from other denominations and traditions, made a considerable contribution to expressing on one hand the pain and loss of those who had suffered, and on the other, the need for community solidarity and for empathy with those who were suffering. Some clergy were simultaneously providing support to bereaved families and those who were injured, involving in some circumstances, very significant commitments, and were centrally involved in planning, ministering and providing pastoral support around the funerals of those who had been killed.

Another important sector was local government. Under the leadership of its chief executive and chairman, Omagh's District Council, the local political authority, provided a forum for political debate and expression in response to the bombing, and mobilised the resources and capabilities of its various departments. This was, at times, very challenging not least as there were political tensions within the Council about the bombing and the rationale behind it. There was also a conversation taking place between local politicians and regional or national politicians. For example, it was brutally clear to most local politicians what the political implications were of the bombing, particularly in the context of the Belfast Agreement, to the question of the legitimacy of violence. These insights informed the advice provided by local politicians to regional political parties and political leaders. In such a challenging environment, the council officers mobilised and delivered its services, including supporting the planning and crowd management of major public events at short notice. The Council also supported the establishment and running of the Omagh Fund, maintaining civic links with the community of Buncrana in County Donegal and with the families in Madrid.

As already noted, the education authority, led by its chief executive and senior managers, played a key role, as did the local schools. The links between the schools and the Community Trauma and Recovery Team were very important, especially in the first 12–18 months when many referrals were received in respect of children, young people and families. Local trades unions, employers and the business community played key roles at times, particularly in underlining the need for solidarity and in identifying themselves with the desire for peace. Additionally and importantly, other public and non-public bodies and disciplines played their part in responding to the needs of the community and in contributing to the various consultations and plans. Those whose work often goes unseen or unnoticed played their part in supporting those directly affected by the tragedy and in contributing to solidarity. For instance, local undertakers, who were almost overwhelmed by the demands made upon them; taxi drivers, many of whom worked with little rest in the first few days after the bombing, often with little or no payment; and the thousands of invisible acts of generosity by neighbours and those who serve the public. Such commitments and acts of kindness were instrumental in binding the community together and, for many, made all the difference at a time of unrivalled distress and difficulty.

The work of the Community Trauma and Recovery Team

From the outset, the Community Trauma and Recovery Team took an open door policy to access. Individuals were not required to be formally referred by another frontline or primary care service. People could refer themselves or be referred by, for example, other family members, family doctors, clergy or the local mental health services. All such contacts were accepted, and appointments offered as quickly as possible. Whilst generally and increasingly people were seen at the centre from which the Team operated, in the early days initial contact with those who had referred themselves or had been referred was sometimes through home visits or telephone calls.

When individuals with concerns or problems made contact with the Team, the approach was to identify and understand their needs through an initial assessment. This usually took the form of a conversation involving a member of the Team. If their needs were not relevant for other services (to whom they would otherwise have been referred with their consent), a more detailed mental health and social assessment was undertaken, sometimes with support from the psychiatrist, art therapist, family therapist, social worker or occupational therapist who were part of the Team. Occasionally additional assessments were sought from other services and disciplines outside the Team.

Routinely, links with family doctors were established and maintained unless a person seeking help wished otherwise – which was rarely, if ever, the case. Once a picture was established of the person's needs they were then signposted to the most relevant member of the Team for psychotherapy or practical services. Before the trauma-focused CBT service developed (described further below) those assessed as having post-traumatic stress disorder (PTSD) or other trauma-related disorders were usually referred to either a counselling or psychotherapy practitioner in the Team, or, if required, to a practitioner in the wider mental health services. From a very early stage, routinely, those receiving psychotherapy or trauma-focused CBT were asked to complete standardised trauma and mental health scales or tools to support the assessment of their needs, to track their progress and to assess their state of recovery when therapy ended. The findings from these assessment tools informed the agenda for therapy agreed between the therapist and the person seeking help.

The team played a key role in maintaining links with the bereaved, injured and others caught up in or adversely affected by the bombing. For example, it was largely through the Team that media interviews with the bereaved and others affected by the bombing were coordinated. This came about because some people, due to their loss, injuries or other circumstances, were much featured in early coverage and felt overwhelmed, wishing to do fewer or no more interviews. Others, who early on were reluctant to do interviews, felt more able to do so as time moved on. In the spirit of recognising the community-wide impact of the bombing, the Team sought to ensure that the widest possible opportunity was created for those affected by the bombing to talk with the media. Likewise, many of the numerous offers of help and gifts from the public were coordinated through the Team, with the support of a designated senior manager from the Trust who managed all offers of help and support to the hospital and community services. This was done largely through a regular bulletin, which was issued by the Team to those who had been bereaved and injured by the bombing. The bulletin was also one of the means by which the findings of the various community needs-assessments (see Chapter 3) were shared.

Very shortly after the bombing a number of bereaved family members formed a self-help group. Its aims initially were to represent the views of bereaved families. The group was accommodated by the Sperrin Lakeland Trust, in offices adjacent to the Omagh Community Trauma and Recovery Team. In the following two to three years, liaison with the leaders and members of the family group played a key part in shaping the developing services and in explaining the impact of the bombing to key agencies and the wider public. Key events, such as the Coroner's Inquest into the deaths caused by the bombing, were discussed and support arrangements determined and agreed between the self-help group and the Team. What became the Omagh Support and Self-Help Group in time moved on to address wider issues related to the bombing, including security and the response by the authorities in Northern Ireland and the Republic of Ireland (Orde and Rae, 2016). In a rare example of its kind, with the lack of success in securing criminal prosecutions, the group took a civil legal action. An account of the group's work and journey was authored by Dudley Edwards (2009).

The development of a trauma-focused therapy service

Understanding the needs of people affected by the bombing was central to the development of therapeutic services by the Team. Key to this was the experiences of those who had been affected by the bombing. In the early weeks the Team heard numerous accounts of those experiences and their consequences, often witnessing great distress, anxiety, anger, withdrawal of engagement in various aspects of life, and the deep concern of family and friends. People spoke about how they felt overwhelmed by their experiences, or how frightened they were, or how they re-experienced images, sounds and smells and bodily sensations associated with their experiences on the day of the bombing, often with powerful emotional reactions. Others, such as clergy, teachers, health practitioners, who were witnessing these emotions, thoughts and sensations in the lives of people they were in contact with, shared similar concerns about those they were supporting. Over time, whilst the number of individuals expressing these things reduced, the intensity and complexity of the difficulties of those who were seeking help later, grew. The difficulties became more elaborated in more striking accounts and complex psychological reactions, often accompanied by feelings of embarrassment that they should think or feel such things, or shame that they were not coping better.

The challenge was to find an approach for making sense of this in ways that were meaningful for those who were having difficulties. Likewise, the approach had to enable those responsible for developing and delivering services to respond appropriately and effectively to people's needs. The team became more precise in its understanding of what people were experiencing and in determining how best services might be of help. The concepts of psychological trauma and of loss became central to understanding people's needs. The risk of those affected by the bombing having or developing mental health disorders was also a major consideration. Specifically, the diagnostic framework offered by PTSD proved to be a very helpful tool for understanding the needs of individuals and in engaging meaningfully and therapeutically with those who were experiencing difficulties. Used flexibly, this also allowed for people who did not meet the full PTSD criteria to receive help from the Team, as an understanding of their needs as trauma-related was key to providing them with help.

Beyond the efforts to better understand the problems faced by those seeking help, there was also the need to develop meaningful and clear therapeutic goals, for the service as a whole and also for each person who was seeking help. Within weeks of the bombing, and on the initiative of the psychiatrist and cognitive therapist leading the clinical service development within the Team, contact was made with a research team based at Oxford University, England, under the leadership of Professor David Clark. The timing of this contact was most opportune in that Professor Clark and Professor Anke Ehlers, plus other colleagues, had just completed work on the development of their trauma-focused cognitive therapy model (Ehlers and Clark, 2000). The Oxford team provided training in their trauma-focused therapeutic approach in Omagh, for the practitioners from the Team and staff from the publicly funded mental health teams – with supervision being provided by video conference. Additionally and importantly, the Oxford team's visits to Omagh included briefings to key public figures and senior staff within a range of agencies about the therapeutic developments at Oxford, and their implications for the therapeutic and service needs of people affected by the Omagh bombing. This contribution was central to the managerial decision by the Sperrin Lakeland Trust to provide a dedicated trauma-focused response to the bombing.

Besides providing orientations to practitioners at an early stage in the development of therapeutic services, the Ehlers and Clark (2000) model provided research-based insights into three important questions, which had implications for the development of services.

1. What are the active psychological components of trauma disorders such as PTSD?
2. What psychological and behavioural responses maintain the trauma disorder?
3. How then can we use trauma-focused therapies to address the components of trauma and the unhelpful psychological and behavioural responses, to overcome and recover from the trauma disorder?

This provided a theoretical framework within which managers and practitioners could operate. The framework was pivotal in imagining what services ought to be developed to address the needs arising from the bombing and in providing clarity on service and treatment goals. The contribution of the Oxford team was transformational in its timing, relevance and in providing a real alternative to a previously unformed understanding of trauma disorders and unclear objectives of trauma services. Within a relatively short time-frame, it moved practice and service aims from merely managing and easing psychological distress, or at best hoping for recovery by providing support, to a position of expecting therapy-aided recovery. At a later point, an audit of therapy outcomes for trauma-focused CBT was undertaken by a partnership of the Omagh team and the Oxford team. The findings demonstrated that no client had deteriorated by the time therapy concluded and that all had made progress (in terms of trauma symptom reduction), with some making very marked progress (Gillespie et al., 2002).

The pattern of demand for trauma support

As noted already, very soon after the bombing and over the following weeks and months, people with emotional, psychological and mental health difficulties began to seek help. The key points of contact were the family doctors services, the local available not-for-profit organisations and the Omagh Community Trauma and Recovery Team. The Sperrin Lakeland Trust's mental health services for both adults and children were also being contacted, mainly by people and families already known to these services. In addition the police family liaison services and the hospital and community services involved in the care of those who had been injured were identifying mental health related difficulties and were referring people to appropriate services. The Trust's occupational health service established on-going contact with the Team both to maintain liaison on the unfolding and changing needs arising from the bombing and to ensure that health and social care staff who needed help, could be readily referred to the Team.

Over the course of three-and-a-half years following the bombing, the

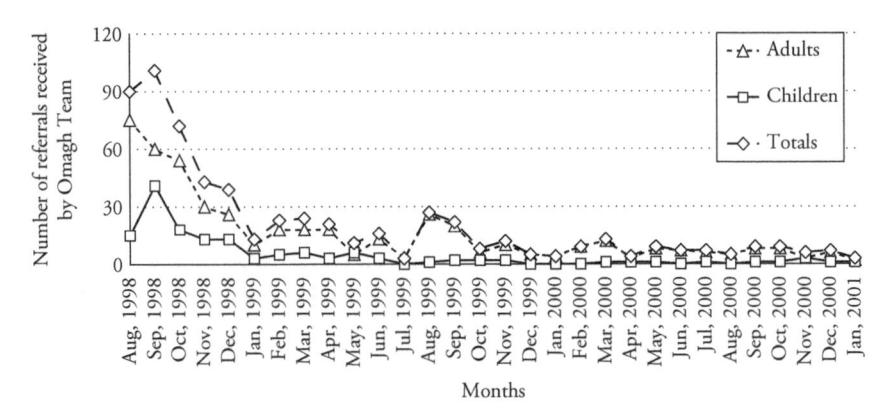

Figure 1: Illustration of the pattern of referrals to the Omagh Community Trauma and Recovery Team, over two-and-a-half years, from August 1998

Community Trauma and Recovery Team received almost 600 requests for assistance, either directly from members of the public or by referral from family doctors, local clergy and faith leaders, District Councillors, other counselling and support organisations, employers and concerned neighbours and friends. The pattern of contacts and referrals over the first two-and-a-half years is illustrated in Figure 1. This shows a relatively high demand from the public in the first two to three months; thereafter demand reduced, with spikes connected to key events until the first anniversary. Following this, there was a low level of demand which continued more or less until the Community Trauma and Recovery Team closed in 2001, just over three years after the bombing.

The nature of the needs expressed in the first two to three months were mainly acute distress, along with concerns from, for example, parents regarding their children, and requests for practical help in relation to education, employment and loss of income. Towards the first anniversary, the nature of referrals changed to more established trauma reactions, including PTSD and trauma-related depression. Thereafter, help was sought in relation to increasingly complicated trauma-related needs. These needs were often associated with daily living problems, such as difficulties in participating in education or employment, family relationship problems, or alcohol dependency.

It is noteworthy that children's referrals declined to near zero by the first anniversary. It is not clear why this was so, especially as there were fewer not-for-profit organisations offering trauma therapy for children and adolescents, but a number of factors might explain this. First, a lot of effort went into raising awareness within the education system of the likely impact on children and young people. The education authority invested much effort in this regard and assigned a senior officer to act as the focal point for schools in relation to needs arising from the bombing. At an early stage the authority secured the support of an independent body to advise it and undertake preliminary work in the first few months with schools and teachers (Pittman, 2000). The Community Trauma and Recovery Team itself undertook a lot of work in support of schools. Then there was the awareness raising created by the Children's and Adolescent's studies (see Chapter 3), undertaken after a lot of consultation with parents and schools. Finally, the child and adolescent mental health team of the Sperrin Lakeland Trust were receiving referrals from an early stage and, with additional resources, developed a capacity to respond to the needs of children affected by the tragedy. On reflection, it would seem that the well-being of children and young people cannot be assumed without acknowledgement of what has happened, without the creation of an expectation of coping along with the appropriateness of asking for help, and the support of important adults who themselves are modeling appropriate responses and coping strategies for dreadful experiences. With some caution, where adults are supported and equipped to identify and address their children's needs and to understand the impact of their own distress on their children, it might also be concluded that children can be more resilient or adjust more successfully.

In establishing the Community Trauma and Recovery Team as a clearly identifiable and symbolic entity, there was a danger of this being seen as the sole focus for responding to the needs arising from the tragedy, and for other organisations, individuals and sectors being either deskilled and immobilised, or 'taking a back seat' in addressing the impact. This was the subject of on-going consideration and many of the structures and liaison arrangements that were put in place were intended to ensure that the Team's work remained a part of a wider engagement, acting as one specific focal point and in support of others. Whilst the Team was often called upon to take a lead on certain issues or was expected to do so, there were times when it was more fitting for others to do so. So for example, at times the churches and faith communities were the appropriate focus, the not-for-profit sector, the District Council, the education authority, the police service, or the health and social care services provider. Sometimes it was obvious who should take the lead, given the needs, purposes or objectives. On other occasions, the lead role was undertaken after discussion amongst agencies and sectors. Ultimately there was a tacit working understanding that from time to time each individual affected by the bombing had different and changing needs, and that it was more than desirable that the community found different voices or ways of acknowledging, expressing and responding to those needs.

Therapeutic challenges

Whilst there was widespread local, national and international support for those affected by the Omagh bombing, there were a number of circumstances which made the seeking of help and the delivery of therapeutic services challenging.

One of these was the number of bomb scares in Omagh after the bombing. For the twelve months following the bombing, on more than a weekly basis, warnings were received of bombs in the town centre or nearby, which at times led to the evacuation of parts of the town. Apart from being very disruptive, this had an adverse psychological impact on many in the community and in particular many of those who were already struggling with their experiences of the original explosion. The Community Trauma and Recovery Team received referrals and requests for help directly in relation to these events. The bomb scares also interfered with help-seeking and engagement in therapy, undermining the confidence of individuals to engage in or continue with therapy.

The bombing had been a political watershed, resulting in political parties clarifying their positions on politically motivated violence in the context of the Belfast Agreement (1998). However, spokespersons for political parties close to the organisations that carried out the bombing, to one degree or another continued to make the case for dissent from the political agreement and others advancing the further use of violence for political ends. One of the challenges therapeutically was to try to support people in these circumstances, where such positions were viewed as unsympathetic, hostile and incomprehensible in the light of the terrible human consequences of the bombing.

Finally, for many of those who were very seriously injured, uncertainty about the future and the need for recurrent surgical interventions and treatment, perpetuated the traumatic event over many months and years. This had major implications for some, and was at times highly disruptive of participation and progress in therapy.

These challenges point to the need to understand and address trauma-related reactions and disorders in the context of the person seeking help, noting that current personal circumstances, along with external events and conditions impact on the ability to engage therapeutically, with implications for the goals of therapy. And as will be discussed later, living under threat (a sense of which the above examples of circumstances induced in many) has implications for the therapeutic task and aims.

Caring for the Team

The flux, the uncertainty and unpredictability, the levels of emotion and distress of those seeking help, and the significant public profile that surrounded the trauma Team did not suit everyone as a place in which to work. The Team, its manager and clinical leaders, the senior management and occupational health services were concerned about the possible adverse impact of working in these highly demanding, therapeutically challenging circumstances in which, of necessity, staff would be exposed to traumatic narrative and content. Significant importance was placed upon supervision and an external agency with extensive experience of delivering therapeutic services in Northern Ireland was invited to lend its support to the Team. Training and support were also important and valued features of staff care. Various measures were put in place, which included personal 'time out' and Team away days, limits on the duration of participation in the Team, limits on workload, variation of workload and specific staff care responses for individuals. Whilst the work was often demanding, the coherence of a new Team engaged on a valued task that was a distinctive part of the community's response to the tragedy seemed to create its own energy and enthusiasm.

A study by Collins and Long (2003a) reported on the experiences, positive and negative effects and support needs of healthcare workers in the Team. It provided important insights into the qualitative experiences of workers who had been seconded to the Team, often at short notice, and who subsequently returned to their normal role and position. The study tracked thirteen healthcare workers who had volunteered to serve in the Team with assessments at four points over the two-and-a-half years immediately following the bombing (T1=0 months; T2=4 months; T3=12 months and T4=30 months). The researchers found that team spirit, camaraderie, satisfaction at seeing patients recover and feeling honoured at being part of the community's recovery, were the more positive aspects of the experience of working in the Team. Mean scores for compassion fatigue and burnout increased over the first year, with reductions in compassion satisfaction, satisfaction with life and life status. However, only a few reported severe problems. Some who left the Team after the first year, due to problems linked to the work, subsequently reported their problems had subsided.

Respondents reported that the extensive media interest (in the bombing, its consequences and the work of the Team), coping with and containing the anger of some patients and dealing with the content of patient's experiences were the most challenging aspects of the work. Returning to normal duties was also challenging, especially where managers provided insufficient understanding and support to their returning staff members. Notwithstanding the difficulties, only one respondent said they would not volunteer to serve in such a team if the need arose in the future. Effective coping strategies identified by respondents included supervision, team building, humour, and a range of relaxation-based activities and opportunities, social engagement, exercise and complementary therapies. The findings resonate with those of other researchers who have examined secondary traumatic stress and vicarious trauma. The authors made a number of important observations with recommendations for supporting staff working in a trauma service following a major tragedy.

The closure of the Team

After three-and-a-half years, when referrals had fallen to a level that could be managed by conventional services, and by which time those services had developed capability in responding to trauma-related needs, and after extensive consultation, the Team was wound up. The closure of the Team was symbolic of progress by the community in the wake of the bombing. The end of the Team's work, and the wider special responses to the bombing by the health and social care services provider, had been envisaged and planned for from the outset (Bolton, 1998). Key to this step was the assurance to local people that there would be alternative services available to meet emerging needs. What happened thereafter is described in Chapter 6.

3

Assessing the mental health impact of the Omagh bombing

Within months it was very clear that the bombing had been a significant stressor in the life of the community. The implications for mental health and well-being were a matter of concern – but poorly defined, and it was not known what the longer-term consequences would be. To ensure that the right type, amount and duration of services would be in place to address the immediate, medium- and long-term needs it was essential that some assessment was made of the impact and consequences of the bombing. This chapter will outline four major needs-assessments undertaken to better understand the impact of the bombing and the way in which the findings helped in the development of services for psychological and mental health needs.

Reasons for investigating the impact of the bombing

As noted in Chapter 1, estimating the likely impact and consequences of the bombing was a significant challenge. Principally, it was not known how many had been exposed to traumatic experiences and of those, how many had, or were likely to, develop longer-term psychological and mental health problems. Therefore it was not known what types and levels of services would be required to assist individuals and the community. It was known from direct clinical contact and discussions within the community that in addition to the experiences of those on the street when the bomb exploded, witnesses and rescuers had been exposed directly to traumatic scenes, along with a large but unknown number of civilians and healthcare workers at the local hospital, and those based at the temporary mortuary. Families, friends and colleagues of those who had been killed were a specific matter of concern. Further, some individuals had been greatly distressed, for example, by the time it took for them to make contact with missing relatives – who were otherwise unharmed. One way of making progress on this matter was to encourage help-seeking. It was thought that this could be enabled by an open discussion in the wider community about the impact of the bombing so that those who were having problems could see that they were not unusual and could also see that there were avenues for obtaining support and help. Also, politicians and funders wanted informed answers to their questions as to what the needs would be and what services and funding were required.

The context for the Omagh needs-assessments

In the history of the Troubles in Northern Ireland there had not been an incident with a combination of so many deaths, so many injuries and so many exposed to highly traumatic experiences. The scale of this particular event warranted strategic consideration of the likely demands for help from the very large but unspecified number of people exposed to traumatic experiences. The challenge facing local services was how to quantify and represent what the impact would be, particularly in terms of well-being and mental health.

The timing of the bombing, occurring just months after the historic political agreement (Belfast Agreement, 1998) and the report of the Victims Commissioner (Bloomfield, 1998), meant that there was a new policy context and wider public expectations that something would be done. These developments had also created an optimism and expectations about addressing the long-term human impacts of the Troubles.

Within the first week after the bombing the senior management team of the Sperrin Lakeland Trust was handling very direct questions from politicians, civil servants, news reporters, and those who had been bereaved, injured or otherwise affected by the tragedy. Questions about what counselling needs would arise and what services would be available were common themes.

Given these circumstances, it was unlikely and indeed unthinkable that there should be no specific additional response to the bombing. Nevertheless, it was, at times, difficult to have the case for action heard and strategically supported, particularly in the face of a poor evidence base about the nature and scale of the need. Besides the desire, and at times the demand, for action in response to the tragedy there were other interests and voices arguing for the opposite. Some felt that nothing special should be done in response to the bombing and that people should be encouraged to seek help through the normal service channels. They argued that no other major strategic response had been made in relation to the mental health needs of other communities affected by over thirty years of the Troubles; that services were in place and people with difficulties would find their way to those services.

At that time, little was known in research terms about the likely trajectory of need and service requirements of communities affected by the Troubles. Whilst there was a body of research related to the impact of the Troubles (see Chapter 4), there was little local research from which conclusions could be drawn about what the expected level of exposure to traumatic experiences associated with the bombing might be. Even if this could be established, it was not clear what proportion of those exposed to the bombing might develop problems in the short, medium or long term. International research indicated wide variations in levels of mental health problems – from studies following natural disasters where the incidence of mental health problems (specifically PTSD) was relatively low, compared to studies of interpersonal violence, which suggested higher proportions could be affected (e.g. Galea et al., 2005).

One method of undertaking needs-assessments was to seek the views of agencies and individuals working directly with the local population and especially with those directly affected by the bombing. However, earlier local experience in planning for the response to other tragedies associated with the Northern Ireland conflict showed that the impressions formed by agencies and practitioners as to how people were coping could not be relied upon solely as a basis for planning and offering services, as they underestimated the amount and severity of need.

Meanwhile, the work of the Omagh Community Trauma and Recovery Team continued and a body of direct clinical evidence was building up as people sought help from the therapy team (Gillespie et al., 2002). The direct therapeutic work provided a highly detailed insight into the changing needs as the initial phase of help-seeking in the early weeks, characterised largely by acute anxiety and distress, gave way to more complicated and long-term problems. As illustrated in Figure 1 (p. 34 above), the numbers seeking help reduced markedly in the first three months or so, but the severity and therapeutic challenge of those presenting later was more complex. The needs of those seeking help, and the work of the Team, were important sources of information, which pointed to the necessity of further assessing the impact; in due course, this information helped to define the needs-assessments that were eventually undertaken. The experiences of local not-for-profit organisations, family doctors and other services were affirming the conclusions being reached by the Team and contributed to the plans for the needs-assessments.

In the first year following the bombing there were over eighty bomb scares in Omagh. These were caused by people who, for unknown reasons, made telephone calls to the police or other agencies to say that a bomb had been planted in the town and was due to explode. The alerts often led to parts of the town being evacuated and emergency services, including the accident and emergency department of the local hospital that had dealt with the casualties of the original explosion, being placed on standby. No bombs were ever found but the threats were highly distressing and very disruptive to the life of a community attempting to recover from the bombing. The studies were being contemplated whilst these bomb scares were happening, and the sensitivity of many local adults and children to the scares reinforced the necessity of better understanding the community's needs.

Taking these matters into consideration, and after much discussion within the community and the Sperrin Lakeland Trust, it was decided that it would be better to ask people directly about their experiences, what difficulties they were having, and how they were coping with them. Plans were put in place for four community needs-assessments, namely a study of the impact on adults, a two-part study of the impact of the bombing on children and adolescents, and a fourth of the impact on the staff of the Sperrin Lakeland Health and Social Care Trust. The designing of these studies benefited from expert guidance from Universities and specialist centres in Britain, Northern Ireland and the Republic of Ireland. The direct knowledge of local concerns, acquired at first hand from those who were bereaved, injured or traumatised by their experiences of the bombing, informed the studies' aims and designs. This included inputs from the self-help group formed after the bombing, local political representatives, civil servants, church and faith leaders, and the various coordinating groups and committees that had been established in response to the bombing.

The adult needs-assessment

The adult study was undertaken by the Trust with the support of Professor David Clark and his colleagues, based then at Oxford University. The key aim was to gain an understanding of the level and nature of exposure to traumatic experiences and of the psychological impact and risks associated with the bombing. The aim was to inform service plans, in particular the development and delivery of trauma-focused therapeutic services. The study instrument was a questionnaire designed to be completed by individuals. It included sections on basic demographic details, current personal circumstances, questions relating to the nature and degree of exposure to the bombing, and about the physical and socio-economic effects, plus three instruments assessing the psychological impact – the Post-Traumatic Stress Diagnostic Scale (PDS) (Foa et al., 1997), the Post-Trauma Cognitions Inventory (Foa et al., 1999) and the General Health Questionnaire (GHQ) (Goldberg and Williams, 1988). Ten months after the bombing, a questionnaire was sent to each adult in the Omagh district – approximately 34,000. Almost 3,100 responded, providing close to a 10% response. The findings could not be understood as being representative of the Omagh population as respondents self-selected. Nonetheless, participants included those who were directly exposed to the explosion, those who were immediate witnesses, those who had suffered a loss – either through the death of a relative or friend, or an economic loss – those who were 'near misses' (i.e. had been in Omagh prior to the bombing but left before it happened), and those who had no involvement at all. Also, the sizeable data-set provided by respondents represented a significant resource from which conclusions could confidently be drawn.

The data provided evidence of significant levels of exposure to the bombing, and the consequences of this. For example, almost 500 people who were at the scene of the explosion or who were witnesses in the immediate aftermath took

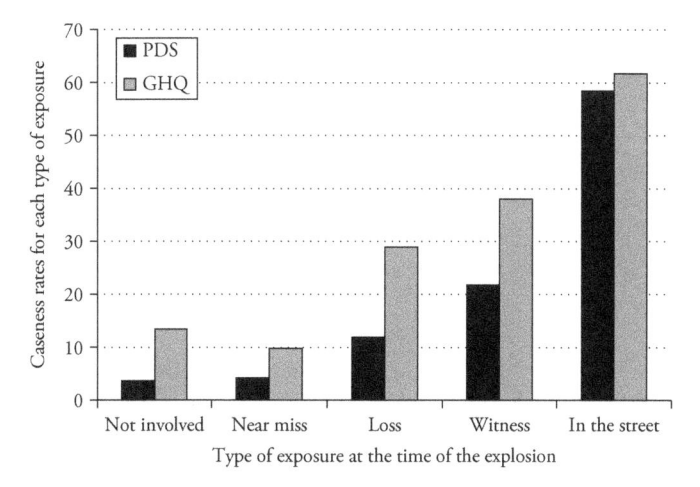

Figure 2: Illustration of the PDS and GHQ caseness levels for adults, for each type of exposure to the Omagh Bombing

part in the study. This was estimated to be over a third of the total who were directly exposed to the explosion or were early witnesses. The findings reinforced the initial assessment, based on observations and conversations, that the bombing was experienced or witnessed by a large portion of the local community, whom the effects impacted upon. The study and key findings have been reported in detail in Duffy et al., 2013.

The psychological impact of the bombing

The findings revealed the psychological impact of the bombing. For example, the levels of probable caseness of PTSD (at 10 months) were 58.5% for those who were present when the bomb exploded, 21.8% for witnesses, 11.9% for those who suffered a loss, 4.2% for the 'near miss' group of participants and 3.6% for those who had no involvement at all. Similar results were obtained with the GHQ (12 item), although being present or a witness were associated with significantly higher PTSD symptom scores (Duffy et al., 2013). These findings confirmed that the bombing had a significant impact beyond those who had been present when the bomb exploded.

The implications for services

In terms of service design and development, the findings on the relationship between exposure and impact on one hand, and the psychological effects, responses and risks on the other, provided a very solid base upon which progress could be made. The results defined what the focus of the developing long-term trauma-focused therapy service should be, and highlighted the significance of cognitions (i.e. how the person was thinking about themselves, others and the world as a consequence of their experiences) in predicting adverse psychological disorders such as post-traumatic stress disorder (PTSD). This was a particularly important finding in that cognitions are amenable to therapeutic interventions. The finding reinforced the direction for the development of services by the Team, i.e. with a particular (but not exclusive) focus on the unhelpful cognitive judgments people with post-traumatic stress problems made of themselves, others and the world in general as a result of their experiences. (See Chapter 7 for a more detailed account of a trauma-focused approach to therapy.)

The role of the media

A majority of respondents felt that the media's role overall was helpful in relation to 'coming to terms with the event' (67%). A small minority felt the media's role was harmful (5.6%). A similar pattern was found in relation to the media's role in explaining the impact of the bombing (77% and 7% respectively). There was an almost unanimous view that the media were helpful in relation to 'providing information about where to get help'. Similar patterns were found amongst those directly exposed to the bombing.

The impact on solidarity

Writing about a disaster caused by the slip of a mining waste tip at Buffalo Creek, Erikson described the loss of communality i.e. 'the network of relationships that make up their general human surround' which was associated with adverse health and social problems (Erikson, 1986: 187). Key drivers included the breakup of settled communities as a consequence of the disaster and the need to accommodate survivors in temporary accommodation as houses and neighbourhoods had been destroyed or where uninhabitable. Erikson described how the disaster had dismantled the social and psychological structures of the very close knit community and identity, and forced people to fundamentally alter their sense of themselves.

One of the aims in the adult study was to ascertain to what degree the bombing might have impacted upon the homogeneity of the community, a concern arising from the political and potentially divisive nature of the attack. The aim was to see if indeed there was such an effect and if so what, if any, associations there might be with adverse emotional and psychological outcomes. Participants were asked to indicate to what degree they felt a part of the community since the bombing. Reassuringly, 53.2% indicated that they felt no different, 40.6% felt themselves to be more a part of the community and only 6.2% felt less a part of the community. When those directly exposed to the bombing were considered on their own, the proportion of those reporting they felt 'more a part of the community', and the proportion of those who felt 'less a part of the community' increased slightly – and statistically significantly.

Spirituality and mental health

To ascertain to what degree having a religious faith or a spiritual outlook on life was in any way protective, the questionnaire also enquired about the degree to which respondents considered themselves to be spiritual. This was relevant in the context of a community where religious practice and church attendance were common. The findings revealed that having a spiritual disposition was neither protective nor did it place the individual at greater risk of developing psychological problems linked to the bombing. This was a valuable finding, as experience had shown that some people who are religious had expectations that they should be able to cope better with their experiences of trauma and loss because of their faith and beliefs. Further, on occasions the expectation of faith communities, fellow believers or family members was that, in view of their religious commitment, individuals should be coping better and not be so distressed. These expectations sometimes gave rise to a further set of difficulties, where for example, the individual questioned the integrity of their faith or their relationship with God. Such reflections sometimes amplified underlying feelings of low self-esteem or shame, or such feelings arising from the experience of the traumatic event.

Asking the question was itself a sensitive matter in a community divided along religious lines and in the context of a tragedy with sectarian overtones linked to those same religious fault-lines. Hence, wording that might be interpreted as asking people what religion they were was avoided, and instead a non-specific question as to whether the respondent 'considered themselves to be a spiritual person' was asked. This part of the needs-assessment was of particular interest to religious leaders and communities with whom the findings were shared and to therapists engaged with individuals for whom religious faith was important.

The findings compare with those of Wilson and Cairns (1992), who looked at how respondents living in Enniskillen following the bombing in November 1987 (the Remembrance Sunday bombing) reported increased church attendance and religious practice, in comparison to respondents from a nearby town that had not experienced as much violence. In this study the focus was on differences in behaviour, whereas the question in the Omagh study was seeking to establish the degree to which spirituality was protective against adverse psychological outcomes of a traumatic event.

Undertaking the adult study and applying its conclusions

This was a major undertaking but the findings were of considerable assistance to the Sperrin Lakeland Trust in shaping and targeting services for the local community. It provided solid evidence of the need upon which advice and guidance on future service developments could be provided to senior politicians, governmental departments and agencies, service commissioners and funders, and the Omagh Fund. The findings were shared with other agencies in the community, such as the education services, schools, not-for-profit agencies and employers.

They were summarised for the two local newspapers through the bulletins provided by the Team to the local community and reported through the monthly meetings of the Sperrin Lakeland Trust. A version was prepared on audio tape for those who had visual impairment. The findings were also shared with services in the Irish Republic that were responding to the needs of the families and community in Co. Donegal and with the Spanish Embassies in Dublin and London.

The findings had immediate implications for the therapeutic services being offered by the Omagh Community Trauma and Recovery Team. They reinforced the trauma-focused approach being taken and led to the further development and refinements of this service, specifically the work of practitioners. In terms of the therapeutic practice of the Team, the findings emphasised the need to make people's thoughts during and after their traumatic experiences a key consideration in understanding and addressing their needs.

The study did give rise to debate. Some people felt it should not have been undertaken and there were concerns that it could upset some. A small number of uncompleted questionnaires which had comments written on them were returned and some of the comments reflected these views. On the other hand, some respondents added positive comments about the study. One bereaved family member complained about the questions relating to the nature of respondents' involvement in the bombing. These were important observations and fair concerns, yet overwhelmingly respondents completed the full questionnaire or most of its instruments. Informal feedback through community contacts suggested that local people greatly appreciated the fact they had been asked about their experiences of the bombing and that they understood and appreciated the reasons why the study was undertaken.

Looking back, the study was a challenging undertaking but was of immense value – not just to the Omagh community but in due course to the trauma therapy field. It was potentially fraught with difficulties and it would have been easy not to undertake it. It was possible because a high level of trust had been established between the health and social care services – not-for-profit and publicly provided – and the local community. It was underpinned by communications before and after the fieldwork was undertaken. Fundamentally, the study was an important needs-assessment following a major traumatic event in the life of a community, one which was intended to be of service to the community. It provided substantial data about need with important implications for planning, service development and practice. Key to its value was the focus on it being a needs-assessment with humanitarian aims, undertaken to assist the community, rather than a piece of research with purely academic purposes. The findings fundamentally shaped the services that were in place and their development in the following years.

The children's and adolescents' needs-assessments

The fieldwork for the Children's and Adolescents' studies was undertaken in November 1999, fifteen months after the bombing, by a partnership of the Sperrin Lakeland's child and adolescent psychiatric services department, the Omagh Community Trauma and Recovery Team, the Centre for Child Care Research at Queen's University, Belfast and Trinity College Dublin, and with the pivotal involvement of the local education authority and local schools. The chief aims were to assess the level of psychological problems amongst younger children and adolescents following the bombing, and, using this assessment of need, to ensure provision of adequate therapeutic resources in response to the tragedy.

Working with the education authority and local schools, arrangements were put in place to inform parents and children of the studies, to seek permission for participation and to put in place the arrangements for the fieldwork to be undertaken. The completion of questionnaires by children and adolescents (8–18 years) took place mainly in the classroom with a member of the child and adolescent psychiatric team or the Community Trauma and Recovery Team present. Twenty-one schools and four training and employment agencies participated in the study, with a combined total of over 4,500 children and adolescents completing questionnaires – out of a total child and adolescent population of nearly 11,500 (from 0–18 years).

The children's study

The younger children's part of the study related to those aged 8–13 years, and in addition to demographic and exposure variables, the main assessment tools were the Children's Impact of Events Scale (Horowitz et al., 1979), the Self Rating Depression Scale for Children (Birleson, 1981) and the Children's Anxiety Scale (Spence, 1998).

The study showed higher rates of PTSD caseness and psychological distress amongst those with exposure to the bombing, plus 'being male', 'witnessing people injured' and perceiving a life threat, as being the most significant predictors for elevated Impact of Events Scale scores. In terms of exposure, the study found a similar pattern of trauma, depression and anxiety symptoms in relation to types of exposure to that described by Duffy et al. (2013) for adults (see pp. 42–3 above). The findings are reported in detail in McDermott et al. (2013).

The adolescents' study

As the second part of the assessment of the impact on children and young people the adolescents' study was likewise undertaken 15 months after the bombing. It focused on young people from 14–18 years attending post-primary schools and skills training facilities. In addition to the demographic variables, Goldberg's shorter GHQ-12 (Goldberg and Williams, 1988) was used along with Foa's

PDS (Foa et al., 1997) and the PTCI (Foa et al., 1999) to assess post-trauma beliefs. An additional set of questions derived from the Ehlers and Clark's (2000) trauma-focused cognitive model were also included. These explored the nature of the exposure to the bombing, the initial emotional response and a set of predictors. The findings are reported upon in detail in Duffy et al., 2015.

The pattern of findings concerning psychological problems in relation to types of direct exposure was similar to that found in the adults' and children's studies. Exposure was associated with higher rates of caseness on both the PDS and GHQ measures. As with the adult needs-assessment, this study provided an opportunity to consider the value of assessing cognitions associated with traumatic experiences and the manner in which the person subsequently coped with their distress and other consequences of the traumatic event. This revealed that the strongest predictors of elevated PDS scores were specific aspects of the traumatic event, what respondents were thinking during the event, and the cognitive mechanisms employed following the bombing. A key conclusion was that the findings supported:

> the suggestion that PTSD in adolescents is primarily associated with their reaction to the specific event, rather than previous characteristics of the young person. The findings ... suggest that exposure alone is not a precise predictor of risk rather it is the aspects of trauma that the young person is exposed to (seeing someone you think is dying); what you are thinking during the event (thinking you are going to die); and the cognitive mechanisms employed thereafter, particularly if a young person develops negative beliefs about oneself, of the PTSD symptoms, ruminates, and the memory retains a sense of the trauma still being in the present. (Duffy et al., 2015: 8)

Follow-up on the children's and adolescents' needs-assessments

Following the needs-assessments, children and adolescents with high scores were identified and their parents contacted for a follow-up clinical assessment involving both a parent (or parents) and the child or adolescent.

This was a complex undertaking, given the sensitivity of engaging with children and adolescents, the need to consult parents and the number of schools and training organisations involved. Also, there was a number of practical and logistical problems in undertaking and completing the study. Despite this, the process of engagement about the study with schools, parents and children seems to have been very useful. It was widely appreciated, helped to raise awareness, and ensured that pathways of help and support were available for children, adolescents, parents and teachers. On the basis of the studies, funding was secured to develop longer-term services for children, adolescents and families.

The health and social care services staff needs-assessment

This study was undertaken on behalf of the Sperrin Lakeland Trust under the leadership of its occupational health consultant in collaboration with the University of Northumbria. The aim was to ascertain the mental health impact of the bombing on staff and to develop appropriate responses and services. The study is of particular interest because it involved an initial assessment (at four months after the bombing) and two follow-up studies (at seventeen and thirty-nine months), hereafter referred to as T1, T2 and T3. The research team produced a number of internal reports for the Sperrin Lakeland Trust (Firth-Cozens and Midgley 1999; Luce, 1999; Luce and Firth-Cozens 2000; Luce et al., 2003) and published a number of peer-reviewed papers looking at different aspects of the study and its findings (Firth-Cozens et al., 1999; Luce et al., 2002; Luce and Firth-Cozens, 2002). The results provided empirical evidence of need and directly shaped the services available to address the impact of the bombing.

The initial T1 questionnaire at four months included the self-report Post-Traumatic Stress Disorder Symptom Scale (Foa et al., 1997) and the GHQ (Goldberg and Williams, 1988), along with questions about respondents' physical health and sickness absence. Staff were asked about their involvement in the bombing response, their job role, what help they had sought in response to any difficulties they had experienced as a result of their involvement and about previous traumatic experiences and psychological difficulties. Copies were sent to all 3,500 members of staff working within the Sperrin Lakeland Trust. The response rate at T1 was 35%, with half of respondents reporting being involved in the response to the bombing. The mean PTSD symptom level scores for those involved in the bombing response group were significantly higher compared to those not involved and were similar to the means scores of witnesses reported in the adult study (Duffy et al., 2013). The highest PTSD symptom levels were associated with having both a personal and professional connection with the bombing, being injured, having someone close killed or injured and being a witness of traumatic events. No gender or age-related relationships with PTSD scores were observed. Previous traumatic experiences were associated with higher PSTD symptom scores (Luce et al., 2003).

The T2 and T3 questionnaires examined the prevalence of PTSD and stress of the respondents and investigated predictors and changes. The mean PTSD and stress scores for 'involved' staff dropped across the three studies. The mean basic PTSD scores for all 'involved' respondents at T1, T2 and T3 were 34.9%, 27.0% and 20.1%, compared with 12.5%, 7.7% and 10.4% for 'not involved' staff (Luce et al., 2003).

Of those who responded, 398 completed questionnaires at T1, T2 and T3 of which 52% had been involved in the response to the bombing. This group had a greater mean age than the original T1 participants, and were likely to have lower

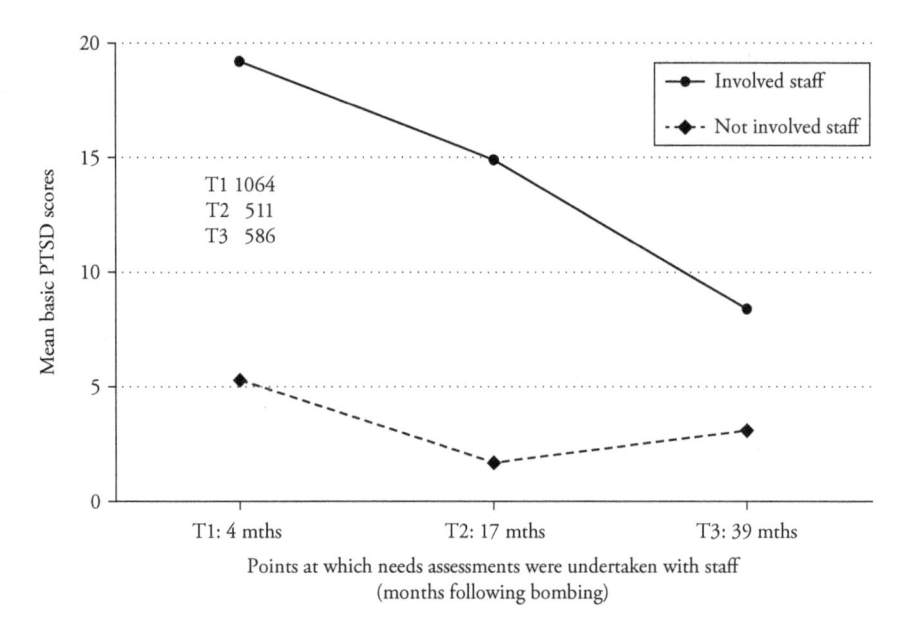

Figure 3: Illustration of the mean PTSD and stress scores of staff involved in the response to the Omagh bombing, compared with scores for those who were not involved

PTSD and GHQ scores at T1. The mean basic PTSD rates for this specific group were 28.4% (T1), 26.4% (T2) and 20.2% (T3) (Luce et al., 2003).

The findings from the staff study were of considerable assistance in understanding the impact of the bombing, in this case on health and social care staff. The findings also drew attention to the impact of a local community tragedy on those upon whom communities rely for their care and support after such events. Those involved in responding to the bombing had mean trauma scores similar to witnesses. The occupational health and welfare arrangements within the Sperrin Lakeland Trust were influenced by the original study (T1), and were maintained and modified on the basis of the evidence from the follow-up studies T2 and T3. The recovery trajectory for the numbers of staff meeting the PTSD level symptoms and the severity of trauma symptoms over the three studies followed the expected path described in the epidemiological study by Kessler et al. (1995). Whilst this gave a sense of concreteness for those involved in determining what services should be provided, over what time period and with what intensity, it also drew attention to the need for early detection of and support for staff (and members of the public) suffering trauma-related disorders. The findings identified the requirement in the long term to ensure there would be access to specialist services for those whose problems had become chronic and encumbered with additional mental health, and other difficulties and disorders.

Conclusions

Within eighteen months of the bombing, the Sperrin Lakeland Trust had the results of four major needs-assessments, which significantly influenced the commitment to the continued provision of services. This formed the basis for making submissions to government for funding. The findings also influenced the direction of service and practice. For example, specific factors, such as unhelpful ways of thinking about oneself, others or the world, were found to be strongly associated with poorer well-being indicators. It was likely these reactions could be addressed through therapy, with prospects of favourable outcomes for well-being. As a result of such findings, high risk groups were identified for whom services could be specifically developed.

Beyond the local benefits, studies that advance our collective knowledge of the intricacies of trauma and that identify the targets for therapeutic interventions are a valuable output. It was always the desire of the chief executive and management board of the Sperrin Lakeland Trust that the knowledge gained from understanding and responding to the Omagh bombing should be made widely available for the benefit of others. The body of internationally available literature on the psychological and mental health risks and service requirements following disasters and conflict that has since become available has increased substantially since the Omagh bombing. In the research literature, the case has been made for trauma-focused interventions to address the psychological and associated impacts of major traumatic events. Governments, aid agencies, emergency planners, service commissioners, service providers and practitioners, and others responsible for responding to major traumatic events have access to significant information and evidence as to the likely needs, the trajectory of those needs and service requirements of affected populations. Further, drawing upon this literature, many national policies, professional standards and academic reviews offer guidance (e.g. NICE, 2005, 2011, 2015). Resources are available, therefore, to guide those charged with responding to the needs of communities affected by traumatic events, and the case for the sort of needs-assessment described above is less pressing.

Nevertheless, further local needs-assessments might be of assistance in given circumstances. For example, all four studies assessed the mental health and related needs of those who were involved in the bombing and those who were not. This provided estimates of the level of exposure to traumatic experiences and helped to isolate the additional impact of the bombing as distinctive stressor. There might be specific characteristics of a particular tragedy that warrant additional research. Cultural considerations or, as in this case, a major event caused by conflict, indicate distinctive local factors on what needs exist and how people might wish to receive help. Such considerations could benefit from additional local assessments. A specific benefit of the Omagh work was the interest many local people took in the studies, which helped to define the needs they could see around them in their community.

Tracking changes in the scale and nature of needs are of particular value, especially when informed decisions about scarce resources are needed. In the staff study described above, there was particular benefit of being able to assess the needs of staff over time, and here again studies to assist in tracking the recovery of an emergency-affected community might be of value. With the availability of computer, tablet and mobile phone systems it has become more feasible to undertake similar studies earlier, to more readily undertake follow-up studies, to do so at less cost, and to minimise some of the concerns by having an opt-in approach rather than paper-based questionnaires arriving in the post.

These studies were very important, both in relation to the Omagh tragedy itself but also as case studies on the implications of the many tragedies that had occurred in Northern Ireland as a result of the Troubles. The studies provided more detail to the available assessments of the impact of the years of violence and contributed important new findings to inform those charged with following up on the recommendations of the Victims Commissioner's Report (Bloomfield, 1998) and the commitments in the Belfast Agreement. The conclusions were verified through the clinical work of the adult and children services working in Omagh in the wake of the bombing. The studies were shared widely within Northern Ireland and, given the enduring needs following forty years of violent conflict, they remain a significant resource for understanding the impact of the Troubles and in helping to define service needs and requirements.

4

The mental health impact of the Troubles, 1969–1999

Northern Ireland's population is approximately 1.7 million. McKittrick et al. (2007) found that 3,720 people had been killed as a consequence of the Troubles between 1969 and 2006. This included killings outside Northern Ireland. In 2010, a study undertaken by the Northern Ireland Statistics and Research Agency for the Victims and Survivors Commission of Northern Ireland estimated that approximately 500,000 people, in Northern Ireland alone, had been affected by the conflict.

> The September 2010 Omnibus Survey found that 30 per cent of the Northern Ireland population had been directly affected by the conflict, either through bereavement, physical injury or experience of trauma (directly or as a carer). The experience of trauma or caring for someone affected by a traumatic experience was reported the most, with 24 per cent of respondents indicating that they had been affected by such experiences. 11 per cent had been bereaved as a result of the Troubles and six per cent have suffered physical injury themselves. (NISRA, 2010)

This chapter provides an overview of the unfolding understanding of the psychological impact of the violence, with reference to key studies, research reviews and other key reports published between 1969 and 1999. In the main, and in view of the weight of material, this chapter focuses on studies and reviews relating to the impact of the violence on adults, although important and broadly similar findings have been found in relation to children through studies undertaken over the same period. The overview reveals that, following a period of apparently little evidence of the impact of the violence on the mental health of the population, it was not until the 1980s that substantive evidence of the impact of the years of violence began to build. Also, research began to reveal something of the dynamics of conflict-related mental health problems. The nature of the evidence, along with the implications of the slowly emerging evidence of the impact of the violence, including the implications for the development of policy and services, are also explored.

The nature of the violence

Throughout the Troubles, for most of the public going about their daily affairs, the everyday experience of the conflict varied from mundane inconveniences to more direct and significant experiences. Commonplace experiences included being searched on entering shops or public buildings, being stopped at checkpoints on roads or being diverted as a result of incidents or alerts. Reading, hearing and viewing media reports on the violence was also commonplace, not least because people relied upon the media to keep themselves informed about possible threats and dangers. More direct experiences included searches of homes and similar operations by the army and police, threats and intimidation, periods of inter-community tension and strife close to one's home, attacks by armed groups or being caught up in major acts of violence such as assassinations or bomb explosions. For those targeted or involved directly in violent events, the impact was likely to involve loss, injury, sometimes threat, extortion, kidnap, torture, exile, and associated psychological distress and trauma, often with significant and longer-term health, emotional, social and economic consequences. Experiences of imprisonment were another potential source of stress, with personal and family consequences. Layered over these experiences was an omnipresent sense of anxiety of varying intensity, made explicit and sometimes amplified by the focus given to particular events. In a relatively small country with a relatively small population, the chances were that everyone knew someone who had been adversely affected by the violence to one degree or another. Besides the Troubles there were the ordinary stresses of industrialised societies. Hewitt (1993) undertook a comparison of the risks of death due to political violence and other causes in Northern Ireland, Italy, Uruguay and Germany. He found that the annual average deaths per million people in Northern Ireland due to conflict was 97.6. This compared with 11.9 for homicide and 179.0 for traffic collisions. The figures for the other two European countries were: Germany 0.1, 40.4 and 251.2; Italy 0.6, 33.7 and 172.3, revealing something of the impact of political violence in Northern Ireland.

Prior to the Belfast Agreement, and by the mid-1990s, ceasefires had been put in place by most of the non-state armed groups (i.e. paramilitary organisations), and the profile of policing, and in particular British Army presence, had been scaled back. The reduction and cessation of violence by armed groups and demilitarisation paved the way for the political talks. However, violence continued up to and following the Agreement. For example, some intra-communal assassinations were carried out, it is generally believed, by groups about to go on ceasefire which seemed to be settling old scores and killing rivals. Post-Agreement violence was carried out by republican and loyalist groups that had not accepted or endorsed the political settlement, or in breach of previously declared ceasefires. Jarman (2004) concluded that from 1996 there had been

6581 sectarian incidents, beatings and shootings, and intimidation. Kennedy (2014) has documented assaults by paramilitaries, misleadingly named 'punishment beatings', on, mostly, young men who had in some way contravened their expectations. Also, street violence associated with protest against and resistance to the perceived erosion of cultural identity or rights, was a feature of this continuing conflict and associated violence. As described in Chapter 1, four months after the Agreement, following a series of major bombings in towns in Northern Ireland, the Omagh bombing was carried out.

The form and approach of Troubles-related research

The form and approach of studies that have investigated the mental health impact of the Troubles varies considerably. The variation has often reflected the opportunities, interests or needs of the researchers or funders. Undoubtedly, the problems of researching a community in civil conflict posed a considerable obstacle for researchers, due to their own anxieties, and the anxieties of individuals and communities that might have been the subject of study. Up until the late 1990s, the majority of studies seem to have been initiated and undertaken by practitioners, service providers or academics working in universities, both in Northern Ireland and elsewhere. From the 1990s, some government departments and agencies, and the Special European Union Programmes Body, have commissioned or funded research. Given the time span involved, the changing nature of the violence associated with the Troubles, the different approaches, group sizes and methodologies used, it is difficult to systematically evaluate the findings over the period. This is particularly the case with post-traumatic stress disorder (PTSD), which was only classified in the 1980s as a distinct disorder, and which has been redefined on several occasions as knowledge grows about the concept. As it took some time for the application of this in local research, there are no early studies, and relatively few more recent studies, which look closely at the disorder. The studies that exist are confounded by the use of different approaches to measuring PTSD. Writing in around 1988, Loughrey et al. note that, 'PTSD is not a diagnosis in common use in Northern Ireland' (1993, 382). Given the distinctive incorporation of exposure to traumatic events or circumstances into the criteria for PTSD, levels of PTSD in a community affected by a major or enuding stressor, such as the Troubles, can act as barometer of the impact of such stressors on the well-being of a community. Its limited use imposes a limitation on the understanding of the unfolding trauma-related needs arising from the Troubles. However, the General Health Question (GHQ) (e.g. Goldberg and Hillier 1979) was used earlier and more frequently and offers a way of assessing the status of groups or the population and of the unfolding impact and understanding of the Troubles.

With regard to the sources of evidence and the types of studies undertaken to assess the impact of the Troubles on mental health, it is possible to identify various forms. These include the following:

- Studies that examine changes in service use, which largely rely upon service use (including pharmacological drugs) or diagnostic statistics available from service providers (e.g. Lyons, 1971; Fraser 1971).
- Clinical studies which look in more detail at small clinical groups of patients or people seeking compensation for their injuries (e.g. Curran et al., 1990).
- Clinical (i.e. relating to counselling or therapy) outcome studies of therapeutic interventions with patients and clients (e.g. Duffy et al., 2007).
- Studies examining in some detail the experiences of particular groups of people affected by the violence (e.g. Grounds and Jamieson, 2002; Lawrenson and Ogden, 2003; Graham et al., 2006; Breen-Smyth, 2012).
- Studies based upon selected samples of the population, groups of people who have experienced violence, and studies based on the experiences in and impact on geographical areas (e.g. Fay et al., 1999).
- Larger community studies examining the impact of particular traumatic events linked to the Troubles e.g. the Omagh bombing series of needs-assessments discussed in Chapter 3.
- Randomly representative population (epidemiological) studies (e.g. O'Reilly and Stevenson, 2003; Cairns et al., 2003; Ferry et al., 2008).
- Meta-analyses summarising the findings from several studies (e.g. Cairns and Wilson, 1993).
- In addition, there have been numerous initiatives and reports providing qualitative evidence of the impact of the Troubles (e.g. Bloomfield, 1998; McDougal, 2007; Ferry et al., 2008; Eames et al., 2009).

Various governmental and non-governmental initiatives have provided opportunities for the receiving of personal and collective experiences of the violence, for instance, The Forum for Peace and Reconciliation (1994–1998, Dublin) and the House of Commons Northern Ireland Affairs Committee of the UK Parliament (2005).

The early years: 1969–1980

One of the earliest studies to investigate the mental health impact of communal violence in Northern Ireland was reported upon shortly after the large-scale violence began (Lyons, 1971). The study focused on three family doctor practices in west Belfast, one of the areas most affected by the early violence. In a sample of 257 patients, identified from either community-based medical practices or from those who had been referred to psychiatrists, there was no increase observed in acute psychotic illness. The researcher found that existing psychiatric facilities were coping with the initial small increase in re-admissions. 'Normal anxiety' reactions were observed in those living in the community, symptoms of which were short lived; in those with a previous psychiatric history the illness pattern usually repeated itself. No increase in the numbers of pharmacological prescriptions, suicides or persons in receipt of social security benefits was detected. Unemployed persons were more likely to develop mental health problems, whereas young and elderly people were less likely to do so.

Another study in the same year by Fraser examined a number of patterns of use of mental health services during the period of civil disturbance in 1969, the summer of which saw the first major episode of violence (Fraser, 1971). He compared the findings to those from the previous year, before the outbreak of intercommunal violence. The key findings were that there were increases in out-patient referrals (for males with psychosis) and psychiatric admission rates (for males with psychosis and females with neurotic disorders) from areas not so markedly affected by the violence – but which might have been considered at risk of more intense violence or attack (referred to as the invasion complex – Fraser, 1973). Whilst there were no changes in referrals or psychiatric admission rates for areas directly experiencing the violence, a significant increase in the prescription rate for tranquillisers was observed. Fraser also commented upon the adverse impact of the violence on children.

During this early period several papers were published, based on studies of mental health diagnoses, suicide and suicide attempts, and on service use. To one degree or another, individual studies pointed to the conclusion that the violence was impacting adversely on the mental health of the population. However, seen against data from wider national and international perspectives, or from innovations in service delivery (e.g. the shift to community-based care) and improved pharmacological interventions, some of these effects had other possible explanations. For example, the apparent drop in suicides in the period 1970–1972 (Lyons, 1972; Lyons, 1979) could be seen in a different light in view of O'Malley's findings of increases in admissions due to attempted suicide (O'Malley, 1972). Later, Lyons and Bindall (1977) set the Northern Ireland findings of falling suicide rates in the context of falling rates in the Republic of Ireland and in Britain over the same period. They did not find that conflict-related violence precipitated suicide attempts.

In his study of mood disorders Lyons (1972) compared the incidence of depressive illnesses in Belfast over two periods – the first covering four years before the outbreak of violence, and the second covering one year following the outbreak of violence. He found that there was a significant decrease in depressive illness in the year after the outbreak of the Troubles compared with the earlier period, most notably amongst men, those over forty years and those in social classes four and five. He attributed the fall in the incidence of depressive disorders to the greater opportunities to externalising aggression. Subsequently, other explanations were explored, including the possibility that the reductions might have arisen as a result of population movements due to the violence, out of the areas under investigation (Darby and Morris, 1974; Loughrey and Curran, 1987; Curran, 1988; Cairns and Wilson, 1993).

Studies relying upon service usage probably faced a number of practical and other problems. For example, there was the possibility that anxieties about street and other violence impacted severely on mobility and therefore on accessing services, including the use of in-hospital services. In comparison to the early studies, which seemed to show little or no significant additional mental health impact of the violence, the later studies (e.g. Cairns and Wilson, 1984; Wilson and Cairns 1992; Daly, 1999; and the later populations based studies such as Bunting et al., 2012) began to reveal something of the additional impact of the Troubles – even where the overall levels of ill-health detected in Northern Ireland were on a par with other nearby countries (the Republic of Ireland, England, Scotland and Wales). As noted, wider changes in health service practices (e.g. the shift from in-hospital to community-based care), along with developments in medication, also seem to be factors in the changing patterns of service use.

The period before the Belfast Agreement: 1980 to 1998

In the 1980s, researchers were noting the lack of empirical research to support an understanding of the impact of the Troubles (Cairns and Wilson, 1984; Wilson and Cairns 1992). One of the earliest studies to use a large community sample to investigate the impact of the violence associated with the Troubles, rather than relying on service usage statistics, was reported upon by Cairns and Wilson in 1984. This involved a sample of 797 respondents from two towns, one of which had, over the previous ten years, experienced high levels of violence; the other low levels. The longer GHQ-30 (Goldberg and Williams, 1988) was used to assess health, and data was sought on perceptions as to the level of violence and safety. Overall, people living in the town that suffered higher levels of violence scored higher on the GHQ-30. Residents from this town who had inaccurately appraised the levels of violence as low, had on average lower GHQ scores (i.e. lower levels of mental health disorders). Those who had high perceptions of violence scored more highly, indicating more accurate appraisals of the level of violence that was associated with higher GHQ scores. The mean GHQ score for women was higher than the mean for men. The researchers concluded that even though there might be objectively high levels of violence, the majority of women coped with this by underestimating the perception of violence – applying the use of distancing, avoidance or denial as means of coping. However, overall the researchers found the levels of pathology as assessed by the GHQ-30 were slightly below the rates derived from studies in Britain in the same period.

An extensive study based on public service diagnostic and service use data by

Murphy (1984) – referenced by Cairns and Wilson (1993) – found no conclusive association between levels of violence and hospital admissions for psychiatric care.

Loughrey and Curran (1987), in an important review of the international literature in relation to the mental health implications of civil disorder, distinguished between studies that investigate early psychological and mental health impacts of civil disorder and later or long-term effects. Studies investigating early reactions amongst people requiring hospital treatment following acts of violence commonly found psychological disturbance, borne out in the Omagh experience (see Chapters 2 and 3). A USA community study by Greenley et al. (1975) found that some who lived in the area affected by rioting felt psychologically better after the rioting. Loughrey and Curran place this finding in the context of the USA in and around 1968 (the civil rights period) and signal its relevance to the link between the wider social and group identity and cohesion, and well-being (i.e. that common group identity and cohesion formed around common social or political aims might be protective of well-being).

Loughrey and Curran reviewed studies from Northern Ireland and other places affected by civil or political violence that had investigated longer-term psychological and related reactions. They found adverse impacts but also what they interpret as evidence of beneficial outcomes in, for example, falls in hospital admission trends. They offer reasons such as: increased social cohesion; the cathartic effects of violent acts; the possibility of late onset masking long-term problems at the time studies were undertaken; and denial and selective migration (i.e. where people having problems leave the areas under study and are therefore do not form part of the dataset).

Loughrey and Curran (1987) were writing at a time when the concept of PTSD was at the early stages of development and had not, therefore, been used systematically to assess patients and trauma-affected populations. They note in particular that, 'PTSD is not a concept familiar to Northern Irish doctors' (p. 14). In an important contemporaneous observation they question the usefulness of trying to compare trauma-affected communities across different experiences and cultures using a wide range of non-trauma specific symptoms and diagnostic categories and without a tool such as PTSD. They conjectured that the category of PTSD under development might provide invaluable if widely accepted and used as a point of reference by clinicians and researchers.

Gallagher (1987) commented upon the focus of research in the early days of the Troubles. He noted a dearth of research, concluding that until 1978 psychologists in Northern Ireland had been reluctant to research the impact of the violence, principally because there was an 'unwillingness to confront some of the social and political issues raised by violence and civil unrest' (p. 21). Early researchers had focused on individual psychological effects and, finding few such effects, concluded that there were few social effects. By contrast, others had reached very stark and extreme conclusions, which in the light of history had proved to be wrong. As a consequence, much of the research that followed therefore highlighted the absence of adverse effects of the violence. Yet, Gallagher noted, in spite of such more optimistic assessments, the conditions and dynamics of the violent conflict in Northern Ireland persisted. He concluded that although researchers were asking appropriate questions (i.e. about the impact of the violence on individuals), they were not asking all the appropriate questions. Prompted by McWhirter (1983), and with reference to Tajfel (1981), he argued persuasively for an approach to the human consequences of conflict using Social Identity Theory, which understands that 'individuals in groups are subject to particular pressures and influences because of and flowing from their membership of social groups' (p. 24).

In 1988, Bell et al. reported on a review of the clinical case records of 499 people affected by civil and terrorist violence in Northern Ireland. The sample included those who were seeking compensation (Muldoon et al., 2005). The researchers found that 4.5% required psychiatric inpatient care, with 11% requiring out-patient services – a total of 15.5% (Kee et al., 1987). They also found that 23% of this cohort had a diagnosis of PTSD (APA, 1987; Kee et al., 1987). The disparity between the proportion requiring conventional psychiatric and related services, and the proportion meeting the criteria for PTSD suggests that levels of use of conventional psychiatric and related services should not be relied upon solely to understand the impact of, and the service requirements of, populations affected by violence. Additionally, in Northern Ireland, psychiatric referrals are usually channelled through frontline services (mainly family doctors); it is therefore likely that a lot of initial distress, and enduring psychological difficulties following traumatic events, are managed by these frontline services without reaching secondary mental health services.

Writing in 1988 about the psychiatric aspects of terrorist violence, Curran concluded that on the basis of usage of psychiatric services, referral and admission data and suicide data, 'the campaign of terrorist violence does not seem to have resulted in any obvious increase in psychiatric morbidity' (Curran, 1988: 473). He offered seven possible explanations. These were: non-reporting; migration; denial (avoidance) and habituation; delayed reactions and onset; the cathartic effects of engaging in or being part of violence; the previously observed beneficial psychological effects of external violence and threat (stress) on those who already had mental health problems; and the cohesive effects of the impact and threat of violence on communities (473–5). Similar effects were noted by Kessler et al. (2006) in their assessment of the impacts of the Hurricane Katrina disaster in New Orleans and surrounding areas in 2005. The researchers noted a rise in the number of people with more serious and moderate mental health disorders yet a fall in suicidality. They found that lower suicidality was related to personal growth following traumatic experiences.

Barker et al's (1988) study, reported in Muldoon et al. (2005), used the GHQ-12 to assess the level of mental health problems in the population of Northern Ireland using a sample of 547 respondents. They found that just under a quarter of the sample had scores above the GHQ cut-off point whereby they could be deemed to meet the criteria for caseness in psychiatric terms. The incidence of caseness was slightly below similar studies undertaken in Britain.

In an extensive review of the research reported upon from the early 1970s until around 1988, Cairns and Wilson (1993) reached a number of conclusions. They provided a critical assessment of early studies and, agreeing with Heskin (1980), pointed to the methodological weaknesses of these studies. They noted the difficulties for researchers seeking to establish the additional impact of the conflict-related violence in the absence of baseline (i.e. pre-Troubles) studies and relying upon small samples. The community studies (which drew upon larger random or representative samples) provided a better quality of evidence. Cairns and Wilson noted in particular that these studies 'added the important proviso that how an individual *perceives* the violence in his or her neighbourhood may be an important factor, interacting with actual levels of violence' (Cairns and Wilson, 1993: 374). They concluded from the body of research 'that only a very small proportion of the population (adults and children) not involved in the civil violence of Northern Ireland have become psychiatric casualties as a result of the political violence' (p. 374). The inference was that those who directly experienced violence were at the greatest and almost exclusive risk of suffering adverse consequences. They noted the evidence from the reviewed research, which indicated that other social stressors, such as unemployment and financial hardship, had a greater impact on health. They concluded that the population had coped well with the stress of the violent conflict, but that 'research has not made clear how this has been accomplished' (p. 374). Quoting Heskin (1980) they identified important enquiries for future researchers: is the coping process masking an inestimable strain?; and is there a latent effect related to the process of coping and adapting to the stress of communal violence and turmoil that will not become apparent until the burden of coping is lifted?

Another study to use the GHQ was reported on in 1990 (Curran et al., 1990). In a relatively small sample of patients (26) seeking compensation for injuries caused by the Enniskillen Remembrance Sunday bombing of 1987, the researchers found high levels of PTSD. At 6 months post-bomb, 50% had developed PTSD. All patients in the sample had high GHQ scores.

In the following year, Cairns and Wilson (1991) reported upon their study wherein they examined three components: (1) self-reported physical health; (2) reported use of family doctor and other health services; and (3) perceptions of Troubles-related violence. They identified an association between perceived high level of violence in the locality where respondents lived and higher numbers of self-reported physical symptoms. However they did not find an association between perceived levels of violence and use of health services. These findings suggest that, again, changes in service usage might not be an appropriate basis for determining need or service requirements of a community in conflict, as noted in Daly's review of the literature (1999).

As a follow-up to their 1984 study (see above), Wilson and Cairns (1992) compared the mental health levels with perceptions of violence in Enniskillen eighteen months after the Remembrance Sunday bombing (November 1987). They found that whilst the majority of respondents in Enniskillen appraised the level of violence accurately, they used less distancing, instead relying more upon cognitive and social strategies, which in turn were associated with increased church attendance and religious practice. Having reviewed the findings from a number of studies, they observed that variations in levels of violence and levels of psychological disorder across Northern Ireland were linked. Yet when other factors had been controlled for, violence only accounted for 'a small proportion of the variation' (Wilson and Cairns, 1992: 349). Where violence was chronic but not particularly prominent, then people were using protective strategies such as distancing, whereas in areas with significant violent events where the denial of violence was unsustainable, then other coping strategies (such as those found in the Enniskillen study) were being used.

To ascertain the workload for a new community mental health team located in a relatively rural part of Northern Ireland (mid-Ulster) Allen, Cassidy and Monaghan (1994) assessed new patient referrals to the team in 1990–1991, excluding those involved in litigation. Of a total sample of 244 family doctor referrals they found that the needs of 8.2% were solely and directly related to the Troubles. Had litigants and those with problems in addition to those with exposure to conflict-related violence been included, then the impact of the Troubles would have been greater. The researchers concluded that even though the area it served was rural and had suffered intermediate levels of violence, the Troubles had 'substantially increased the ... team workload' (Allen et al., 1994: 67).

In 1997, the health department of Northern Ireland noted in its regional strategy that 'Many (people who have been bereaved or injured) have been traumatised by violent events but have yet to be identified as victims'. The strategy was targeted towards people, groups and areas objectively shown to be in greatest social need, and set out the ambition of ascertaining 'systematically the extent of current needs of this group of people and the most appropriate ways of responding to them' (DHSS, 1997; cited in DHSS, 1998: 3).

The Cost of the Troubles Study: 1998

Following the main paramilitary ceasefires in Northern Ireland in 1994, a group of people from all sections of the population in Northern Ireland who had direct experience of bereavement or injury in the Troubles was formed to discuss their contribution to the developing political situation. A limited company and charitable body called The Cost of the Troubles Study was created, comprising academic researchers, people working in communities, and some who had had personal experiences of violence. The intention was to undertake a two-year project in line with participatory action research principles which would, amongst other things, examine the nature and prevalence of the effects of the Troubles-related violence on the general population of Northern Ireland. Some of the specific aims were to produce:

- a mapped distribution of deaths during the Troubles;
- an exploration of the relationship between deprivation and the geographical distribution of deaths in the Troubles;
- a measure of prevalence, extent and diversity of the effects of the Troubles on the general population of Northern Ireland;
- a measure of the extent and range of services used by those affected by the Troubles, and their evaluation of those services. (Fay et al., 1998)

The study produced the first in a series of reports in 1998. The researchers provided a detailed account of the pattern of violence across Northern Ireland, relying largely on proxy evidence, that is, the relative levels of violence were inferred with reference to the number of Troubles-related deaths in local government areas. They also reported on the experiences of those upon whom the Troubles had impacted. In relation to mental health they concluded that almost 30% of those who participated in the study, and who had been exposed to violence associated with the Troubles, had needs approximating to PTSD. The mental health measures used in the study mean that the findings are difficult to compare with those of other studies, and the levels of mental ill health and PTSD are probably an over-estimate (McWhirter, 2004). Nonetheless, the study is an important contribution to the efforts to understand the impact of the violence. It established links between the levels and intensity of violence and deprivation. The study found an association between how much respondents felt the Troubles had impacted upon them and health status, with areas of high intensity violence having worse health profiles, and vice versa. The study also provided estimates of the deaths and the organisations that were responsible for them, which in the context of the developing peace process was a valuable perspective on the historic past.

Prior to the publication of the study, the project director made a submission, commenting upon needs the research team had identified, to the Victims Commissioner (Bloomfield, 1998) as he was preparing his report.

> One study we conducted showed that roughly 50% of people still had symptoms of emotional distress and things like sleep disturbance over 20 years after they had

been bereaved in the troubles. This means that the scale of the problem may be very large. If we count only immediate family members, there could be over 41,400 people in the population whose immediate family death or injury in the troubles has directly affected, and who suffer distress or emotional disturbance as a result. This figure does not include all the eyewitnesses, neighbours, friends, extended family, co-workers and so on who have been affected by deaths and injuries in the troubles. (Smyth, 1997: para.12)

This was one of the earliest attempts to quantity the numbers of people within the population who might have mental health needs relating to the Troubles. The project director also commented upon current policy and service provision.

There has been a total absence of public policy in relation to this area, a total lack of professional training and very little or no support for initiatives in the voluntary [not-for-profit] sector. This is partly due to a culture of silence and denial around issues related to the Troubles, which was part of our survival and coping strategies whilst the violence was ongoing. (Smyth, 1997: phase 1: 1)

It was recommended to the Victims Commissioner that an organisation be formed to promote services to those affected by the Troubles. A number of important recommendations were made about how services needed to become attuned to the needs of those suffering physical and mental health impacts of their experiences. There was also an emphasis on the need for further training in relation to psychological and trauma-related needs and the development of expertise in addressing the complex trauma-related needs of adults and children. In view of the aversion to addressing the experiences and needs of individuals and communities affected by the Troubles, Smyth said that public bodies and professional bodies in health and social care should address their cultural orientations and cultures, 'to develop policy and practices which reflect the past and are appropriate to the new situation' (Smyth, 1997: phase 1: 2).

Subsequently, the findings in relation to mental health and other needs, relating to both adults and children, were the subject of a series of reports and other publications and submissions in a form that made them widely available to and accessible for policy-makers, service commissioners and service providers.

The Belfast Agreement: 1998

The 1998 Belfast Agreement was built upon a number of strands of negotiation and an architecture that sought to recognise and equate the national identities and aspirations of the two main traditions, that is nationalist/republican and unionist/loyalist. Within the Agreement the participants committed themselves to 'acknowledge and address the suffering of the victims of violence as a necessary element of reconciliation'. It went on to say: 'It is recognised that victims have a right to remember as well as to contribute to a changed society. The achievement of a peaceful and just society would be the true memorial to the victims of violence' (Belfast Agreement, 1998: 18).

The Agreement also contained the recognition that:

> The provision of services that are supportive and sensitive to the needs of victims will also be a critical element and that support will need to be channelled through both statutory [publicly provided] and community-based voluntary [not-for-profit] organisations facilitating locally-based self-help and support networks. This will require the allocation of sufficient resources, including statutory funding as necessary, to meet the needs of victims and to provide for community-based support programmes. (p. 18)

The Victims Commissioner's Report: 1998

The parties to the Belfast Agreement looked forward to the results of the work of the Northern Ireland Victims' Commission. A commissioner had been appointed prior to the Agreement by the British Government to bring forward a report into the needs of people who had been affected by violence and to make recommendations. The Commissioner's Report (Bloomfield, 1998) was published some weeks after the Agreement. In the light of subsequent findings about needs linked to the Troubles, the report contained relatively little detailed analysis of needs and was substantially a personal synthesis of the extensive consultations undertaken by the Commissioner. The significance of the Commissioner's work and his report lay more in how it brought acknowledgment and legitimacy to the many in the community who had invisibly and quietly suffered as a consequence of the violence, and in particular those who had been bereaved. The report did not meet with universal approval in that for some it was silent or insufficient in relation to some experiences of violence. Whilst it acknowledged the impact of traumatic experiences, proposals on how services might be developed to address the mental health legacy of the violence were limited. However, as a formal government-initiated enquiry into the human impact of the violence, the Commissioner's role and report acted as a counterweight to the technical diplomacy of the political talks and the Belfast Agreement. It established a foothold for victims and survivors as actors in the peace-building and political processes and set the scene for the later development of a Victims and Survivors Commission and Service. The timing, just after the Agreement was reached, was salutary, in that it reminded politicians, some of whom were still wrestling with the question of the legitimacy of violence, and the wider community that when political disagreement becomes violent conflict, individuals, families and communities pay a heavy price.

Living with the Trauma of the Troubles: 1998

Within weeks of the Belfast Agreement, and shortly before the publication of the Victims Commissioners report, the Northern Ireland's governmental health department published a report, *Living with the Trauma of the Troubles* (DHSS, 1998). This was based on the efforts of a working group established in 1987 by the department to 'examine and promote further the development of services to meet the social and psychological needs of individuals affected by the conflict' (p. 6). The working group observed that 'in recent years there has been a growing realisation, both locally and internationally, that individuals caught up in traumatic events can suffer psychological symptoms' (p. 9). This conclusion, rather understated in the light of more recently available data, reflected the low level of public service awareness of the impact of the Troubles at that time (1997–1998). The report noted that 'a proportion of all referrals to … psychiatry and psychology services are related to problems associated with the civil unrest' and that 'Those providing addiction services have found that a significant proportion of people referred can trace their addiction back to events related to the conflict' (p. 9). In their evidence to the working group The Samaritans, a confidential telephone helpline service for people with emotional and psychological distress, revealed that 'a striking proportion of their calls are from individuals have been affected by the conflict' (p. 19–20). The report made observations on aspects of current service provision based on the evidence received from contributors to the working group. For example, access to services was considered by some to be a problem both in terms of geography and waiting times. In the context of civil conflict, contributors also raised issues of trust in public and other services. The report reflected tensions in relation to counselling and support services and concerns around the medicalisation of emotional and psychological problems. It was concluded that those most severely affected by the violence may require specialist help from mental health services, but that in view of the perceived stigma associated with such services, individuals should not be referred unnecessarily. Concerns were also expressed about the use of the term 'victim' in that its use might consign people affected by violence to a passive, dependent status when they may wish or need to be to be actively involved in working towards recovery. In the light of current international knowledge of the risks of traumatic experiences for physical and mental health, some of the report's observations seem dated, if not at times extraordinary. However, it provides a window on the perceptions held within agencies and the sectors representing and involved with victims of the Troubles around the time of the Belfast Agreement.

The report made a number of important recommendations that included proposing a set of principles (p. 23) that should underpin future service development. It included frameworks for understanding and mapping the unfolding needs and service requirements of disaster-affected populations (Gibson, 2006).

Another recommendation proposed that a working party should be established to address the 'widespread concerns about the counselling of persons affected by the conflict' (p. 13) to address issues such as training, accreditation, supervision, coordination, quality and effectiveness. The report recommended that each of Northern Ireland's Health and Social Services Boards, that is, those agencies responsible at that time for commissioning and providing health and social care services within Northern Ireland, should establish a small advisory panel made up of public service practitioners and not-for-profit service organisation representatives, and include people who had experienced traumatic events. The aims of these panels were to assist coordination, to streamline services, to improve the understanding of needs, and to improve service responses. Following the report, all Health and Social Services Boards established Trauma Advisory Panels to take on the functions recommended by the working party.

The development of the self-help victims' and survivors' sector

The Belfast Agreement had failed to secure the support of a significant portion of unionist political opinion and the Democratic Unionist Party demurred from the Agreement. Making peace requires compromises and one of the effects felt by some unionists was that the loss and suffering caused by the campaign of terror, chiefly from republican armed groups, was being discounted by some of the compromises required in the Agreement. This perceived deficit was amplified by comparisons of the levels of funding being spent on prisoner and former prisoner support groups and those representing people who had been affected by the actions of armed groups. This led to the British Prime Minister making substantial funding available within days of the Agreement to address the needs of civilian victims of the violence. This was followed by the formation of more self-help groups and organisations, part of the purpose being to make visible and represent those who had been bereaved and otherwise affected by the violence of non-state armed groups. Dillenburger et al. (2008) estimated that 60% of all victim and survivor support groups in 2006 in Northern Ireland were formed following the Belfast Agreement (Figure 4).

Review of research: 1999

Daly (1999) provided an important reflection on the previous research in the context of the political progress in Northern Ireland and developing knowledge about trauma-related disorders. A psychiatrist working in the public sector, who had an enduring interest in the impact of the violence linked to the Troubles, he noted the limitations of understanding some of the findings from the early research in relation to concepts such as PTSD, which had only been developed in more recent years. He concluded that even though Northern Ireland had (overall)

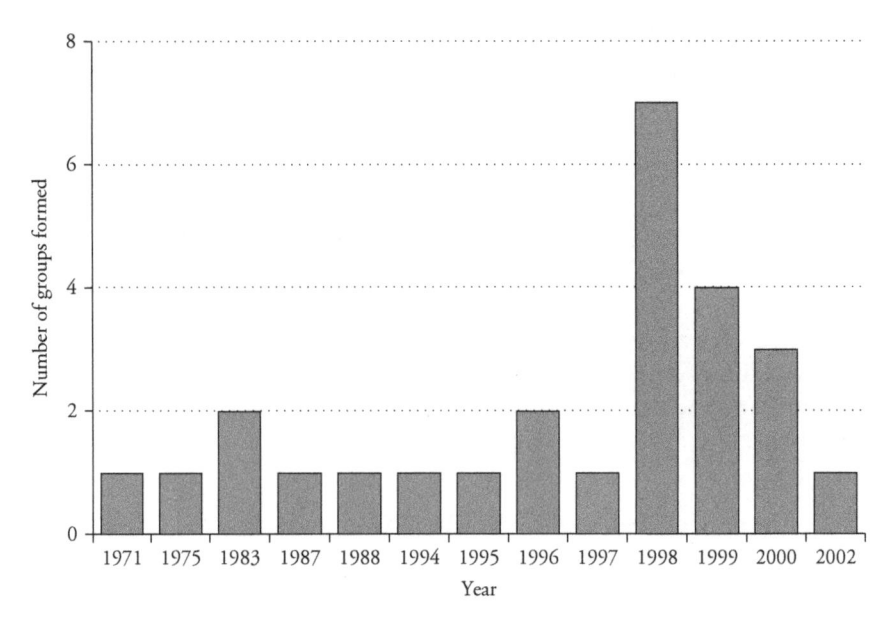

Figure 4: Number of self-help groups formed in Northern Ireland in relation to the Belfast Agreement

a static population, valuable opportunities for research had probably been missed and that the extent of the conflict/trauma-related problems in Northern Ireland remained unknown (i.e. in 1999). Due to lack of familiarity amongst doctors with the concept of trauma and associated disorders he surmised that there was a possibility of under-diagnosis of trauma-related disorders. He described some of the problems family doctor services have in understanding the needs of patients who have been exposed to traumatic events, because they did not know about individual patients' traumatic experiences and loss. This, he concluded, has led to difficulties in estimating the extent of the problem. Much of the progress in understanding the needs of individuals affected by traumatic events linked to the Troubles seems to have been made as a consequence of consultations with psychiatrists with an interest in trauma, who were assessing patients for compensation purposes. This meant that sometimes people seeking compensation had their trauma-related needs identified for the first time through the compensation process. Noting the evidence 'that there may have been more psychopathology secondary to the civil disturbances than many have previously thought' (p. 203), Daly also cautioned against over-diagnosis and medicalisation of post-traumatic psychological reactions that might otherwise be short-term and require little or no psychiatric intervention. He identified the 'need for a detailed epidemiological community study which specifically addresses the issue of trauma, its psychological effect upon the population and the extent of the problems' (p. 204) in the population. Daly noted that 'The Troubles have not had a uniform effect on the population – they have tended to be concentrated upon urban districts, with only a small number of rural areas experiencing major ongoing disturbances' (p. 203). The victims had been predominantly working class. In addition, there had been specific groups of people within the population at much greater risk of being victimised. He identified the security forces, children, the bereaved and prisoners as groups with distinct needs. Daly recommended the formation of a stratified service. This should be largely locally accessible to overcome, amongst other things, the ghettoisation of many communities and groups affected by the violence. It should involve a mixed economy of services provided by public psychiatry and mental health services, not-for-profit organisations capable of delivering relevant and effective services, and with a role for community services such as family doctors, clergy and others in addressing less severe needs. He saw a role for a regional centralised component to this service, which could provide very specialist therapeutic services and training, and undertake research.

Lost Lives – a chronicle of deaths in the Troubles: 1999

In 1999, *Lost Lives*, a chronicle of the deaths associated with the Troubles in Northern Ireland, was published (McKittrick et al. (revised) 2007). The compilers relied mainly on journalistic accounts of deaths, together with material from books, pamphlets and broadcast material, to provide a summary of each death and the circumstances. It was not designed as academic research, and nor did the compilers set out explicitly to measure the health-related consequences, but by merit of its contemporaneous sources and the fact that it brings together accounts of 3,720 deaths, the human impact is revealed in some detail. The book provides evidence of suffering and loss, as well as the personal, social and economic impacts on adults, children and communities. More than anything perhaps, the book illustrates and provides evidence of the significance of the violence associated with the Troubles as a distinctive, significant and enduring stressor over thirty years and more, on the life of the community.

Conclusions

This chapter has examined key studies, along with the works of various groups and authors, to understand the human and psychological impact of the Troubles from the outbreak of violence in the late 1960s until 1999, the year following the Belfast Agreement. The next chapter will review research from 2000 until 2015, ending with conclusions and a commentary on the changing understanding of the impact of the years of violent conflict.

5

The mental health impact of the Troubles, 2000–2015

The long-term impacts of Bloody Sunday: 2000

Hayes and Campbell (2000) provided an account of the political context for the delivery of social care services in Northern Ireland during the Troubles. The researchers examined the experiences of families whose relatives had been killed or injured in the Bloody Sunday shootings of January 1972. Using the framework of PTSD they found high levels of psychological morbidity and some evidence that families had not received services that may have helped resolve their trauma-related needs. They concluded that opportunities to create new services in the context of the developing peace process could provide new ways to address the unmet needs of people adversely affected by the Troubles.

An audit of referrals to a mental health department: 2001

An audit of referrals for psychiatric services to the Mater Hospital Belfast, which continues to serve an area deeply affected by the years of violence and characterised by significant socio-economic and cultural divisions, and deprivation, was undertaken by Curran and Miller. They found that 'only 6% of referrals and admissions had as their precipitants any violence related issues' (Curran and Miller, 2001: 75). Their audit of 2191 persons affected by acts of terrorist and criminal violence found that only 2% were admitted for in-hospital psychiatric care, while 13% were referred to out-patient mental health services or counselling services.

The Northern Ireland Health and Social Wellbeing Survey: 2001

O'Reilly and Browne (2001) reported upon the Northern Ireland Health and Social Wellbeing Survey of 1997 focusing on health service use. They found that 27.6% respondents had a General Health Questionnaire GHQ-12 score of 3 or more and 21.3% had a score of 4 or more. Women were more likely than men to have poor psychological health. Compared with England or Scotland, Northern

Ireland had a higher prevalence of psychological morbidity. Catholics tended to have higher GHQ-12 scores than Protestants.

The Northern Ireland Health and Social Wellbeing Survey of 2001 (NISRA, 2002) explored stressful life events, mental health problems, stress and social support needs in the population. In relation to the Troubles, people who said they had been affected a lot by the Troubles were almost twice as likely to show signs of a possible mental health problem as measured by the GHQ-12 (34%), compared to those who said they had not been affected much (18%). Overall 21% scored highly on the GHQ-12, showing signs of a possible mental health problem. Adults who were affected a lot by the Troubles were more than twice as likely to have experienced a great deal of worry or stress over the previous twelve months, compared with those had not been affected much by the Troubles (22% and 10% respectively) (NISRA, 2002: 3).

The inclusion of the GHQ-12 into the Northern Ireland Household Panel Survey in 2001 for the first time enabled Murphy and Lloyd (2007) to undertake a comparison across the four nations of the UK and 'to assess the impact of low-intensity warfare on rates of psychiatric morbidity in Northern Ireland and to compare these with psychiatric morbidity rates across England, Scotland and Wales' (p. 397). Based on a detailed analysis of the GHQ-12 data for each of the four countries of the UK, the researchers found that the psychological health of people in Northern Ireland was better than those in Wales, and marginally worse but close to those in Scotland and England. The findings are a snapshot, however, and the lack of deployment of the GHQ in earlier studies makes it difficult to assess to what degree well-being in the four countries has improved or worsened, prior to this study.

In a closely argued discussion drawing from the work of a number of researchers, Murphy and Lloyd suggest that in Northern Ireland 'psychological health is damaged in specific geographical areas where there is high violence (and usually high social deprivation)' (p. 403). They draw attention to the patterns of psychological ill health found in their study associated with 'geography, religious identification, gender and/or indices of social deprivation' (p. 403) and suggest that 'rather than assume that the conflict has a global effect on the Northern Ireland populace, inequities in well-being across [Northern Ireland] may be a more plausible explanation for the findings reported in the present study' (p. 403). They acknowledge the different results found by Miller et al. (2003) using a larger sample 'which reported high levels of stress and anxiety in the populace' (p. 403). They offer ways forward for further research and suggest that one area of future study (building upon Cairns' and others' deployment of Tajfel's Social Identity Theory) is to consider that 'The appraisal and subjective meaning of the person's experience may be pivotal in the effect the conflict will have on indices of psychological health' (p. 403).

The article by Murphy and Lloyd is interesting in that it seeks to disentangle apparently conflicting observations and conclusions that on one hand the Troubles have not had a global adverse effect on the well-being of the population of Northern Ireland, and yet that other studies and clinical practice demonstrate that individuals are indeed adversely affected by their experiences. Investigation of the role played by the appraisals and subjective meanings that people have of their experiences and circumstances might contribute to understanding why later studies report a much greater impact of the Troubles (as politics took hold) compared to earlier studies (setting aside some of the methodological differences). This is discussed further below and in Chapter 9.

Mental health and unmet needs in Derry/Londonderry: 2002

In 2002, McConnell et al. reported upon their epidemiological study of mental health disorders and needs for treatment of the general population (aged 18–64 years) in the city of Derry/Londonderry. One of the instruments used to assess those who responded to an initial postal questionnaire, and to select them for clinical interview was the GHQ-28 (Goldberg and Hillier, 1979). Of 1088 returned questionnaires, 304 (27.8%) scored 5 or more on the GHQ-28. Based on a single diagnostic category (i.e. not counting those with more than one disorder) the twelve-month prevalence of mental disorders (as defined by the 10th revision of the International Statistical Classification of Diseases and Related Health Problems – ICD-10; World Health Organization, 1992) was 12.2%. The researchers concluded that the prevalence for depressive episodes for Derry/Londonderry was greater than the UK average, and overall the prevalence of psychiatric disorders was similar to a deprived inner-city area of London. In terms of treatment, the researchers found that, 'While 71% of meetable needs for depression had been met, only 19% of those relating to anxiety were met. Thus anxiety disorders were under-treated, even though they were often long standing' (p. 218). The numbers for individual disorders were generally too low to allow conclusions as to the prevalence of such disorders in the community under study.

Whilst mindful of the Troubles and relative deprivation of the population under study, the researchers did not report upon the level of exposure to Troubles-related or other traumas.

The Omagh bombing studies: 1998–2002

As described in Chapter 3, the bombing in Omagh (1998) gave rise to a number of studies and the availability of data on needs and the impact. The Omagh studies and service data comprise a multi-dimensional longitudinal community study in the context of the Troubles, undertaken over three-and-a-half years. This commenced with the early community studies (e.g. Firth-Cozens, et al. 1999; Duffy et al., 2013, McDermott et al., 2013; Duffy et al., 2015). There then followed data derived from the flow of information from service providers (see Chapter 2), and the study concluded with the work undertaken by the Omagh Community Trauma and Recovery Team on the outcomes of an audit of a trauma-focused therapeutic service for PTSD (Gillespie et al., 2002).

Gillespie et al. (2002) carried out an audit of therapy outcomes for 91 patients with PTSD who attended the Omagh Community Trauma and Recovery Team and showed significant symptom reductions (see Chapter 2). The researchers reported upon the trauma-related mental health needs and therapy outcomes of patients affected by the Omagh bombing: 76% were assessed as having chronic PTSD and 24% as having acute PTSD. Of the 91 patients, 70 were female; 33% had been physically injured by the bomb explosion; 42% had been present but not injured; 12% were staff of emergency organisations who attended the scene or treated people in hospital; 54% had one or more co-occurring mental health disorders, as well as PTSD. Patients were assessed using the Post-Traumatic Stress Diagnostic Scale (PDS) (Foa et al., 1997), the Impact of Events Scale Revised (IES-R) (Horowitz et al., 1979), the Beck Depression Inventory – Second Edition (BDI) (Beck et al., 1979) and the GHQ (Goldberg and Williams, 1988). Patients were provided with the number of sessions of trauma-focused cognitive behaviour therapy deemed appropriate to reduce their symptoms to an acceptable level (median of 8). The audit revealed statistically significant reductions in trauma, depression and general mental health scores (i.e. on the PDS, the BDI and the GHQ). The outcomes compared favourably with those from a series of randomised controlled trials for CBT.

The study, and the series of studies it formed part of, provided a distinctive overview of a community affected by the Troubles. This included a baseline picture of the early impact of a major traumatic event in the life of a community and its members and, thereafter, how needs and service requirements changed.

The experiences and needs of ex-prisoners and their families: 2002

In 2003 Grounds and Jamieson reported on the effects of long-term imprisonment amongst 18 republican ex-prisoners and their families. The ex-prisoners had spent an average of eleven years in custody. The researchers heard about 'complex experiences of loss, psychological change and social adjustment difficulties, together with persistent barriers to social integration, particularly in the area of employment' (p. 347). The participants, who were assessed for depression and PTSD, were found to have a range of mental health problems some of which were in the 'severe' category. The study revealed significant personal, social and economic impacts of imprisonment on life following release. Significant challenges and problems were also identified for families, both during the time their family member was imprisoned and following release. Some continued to experience problems for up to a decade following their release.

The needs of ex-prisoners continued to be a difficult subject for many who had experienced the violence, threats or intimation of armed groups (i.e. paramilitary groups). As Jarman (2004) and Kennedy (2014) have recorded, some paramilitary groups attacked people long after the Belfast Agreement was in place. Given the numbers who were imprisoned in Northern Ireland as a result of the Troubles, from a public health and well-being perspective, the needs of ex-prisoners and their families is not insignificant. Rolston (2011) summarised evidence from a number of sources. He found that in the early days of the Troubles, 1,981 people had been interned (Bowcott, 2010). It has been estimated that 15,000 republicans and between 5,000 and 10,000 loyalists were imprisoned (Shirlow and McEvoy, 2008). These figures do not include those held on remand (e.g. before being released with no charges or after being found not guilty). Ex-prisoners comprise a significant proportion of, mainly, the male population. Rolston (2011) notes the striking conclusion by Jamieson, Shirlow and Grounds (2010) that politically motivated former prisoners make up a significant portion of the male population in Northern Ireland. Having extensively reviewed the literature and notwithstanding some detailed studies of groups of ex-prisoners, Rolston (2011) concluded that there was no systematic study of their experiences and the effects the conflict had had on them.

The 1997 Northern Ireland Health and Social Wellbeing Survey: 2003

O'Reilly and Stevenson (2003) examined the effects of the Troubles by carrying out a secondary analysis of data collected on 1,694 respondents aged 16–64 as part of the 1997 Northern Ireland Health and Social Wellbeing Survey. The data reinforced the association between poor health indicators and adverse social conditions. In examining the likely effect of the Troubles, they found that overall, 21.3% of respondents said that the Troubles had either had 'quite a bit' or 'a lot' of impact on their lives or the lives of their families. The corresponding figure for impact on their area of residence was 25.1%. Analyses of GHQ-12 data revealed that respondents whose lives or areas had been affected by the Troubles were more likely to experience psychological problems. In comparison to this, the researchers found 'a positive and graded relation between the extent to which people and areas were affected by the Troubles ... and the likelihood of suffering from significant mental health problems' (p. 491). They identified the adverse impact on people who lived in areas affected by violence and others, who lived in less affected areas, but whose lives had been affected by direct experiences of violence – an important nuance in understanding the complex impact of the Troubles. Having examined other possible factors and compared findings from Britain and the Republic of Ireland, O'Reilly and Stevenson concluded that, 'the Troubles are a separate and additional burden and therefore contributes significantly to the higher psychological morbidity in Northern Ireland' (p. 491).

As already noted in Chapter 4, several studies have utilised or commented upon the usage of service use data to demonstrate need. In this study, O'Reilly and Stevenson observed that:

> It is however possible that the levels of psychological morbidity were generally increased without an apparent increase in the use of health services or change in trends in national mortality statistics. Many of the indicators of mental health that are largely based on contact with the caring professions will underestimate the impact of the Troubles if there has been significant denial or under reporting of symptoms and there is some evidence to suggest that most people in Northern Ireland deal with the stress generated by the political violence by denying the existence of the violence around them. (p. 491)

In an editorial commenting upon O'Reilly and Stevenson's paper, Kelleher (2003) explored the interplay between historic and contemporary disadvantage and inequalities – and the direct experience of conflict and violence. She discussed their relevance for the relatively poorer mental and physical health profile of the population in Northern Ireland, compared with other nearby regions and countries. Whilst noting the unavoidable significance of experiences of violence for health and well-being, she also explored the degree to which structural and historic disadvantages and inequalities have played a part in long-term patterns of poor health. She made the important point that a range of interventions are required to tackle the individual, group or neighbourhood and population determinants of poor health needs and profiles.

Who are the victims? 2003

In a study commissioned by the Northern Ireland Office, Cairns et al. (2003) found that the mean GHQ-12 measure of a sample of 1000 adults from across Northern Ireland was 10.05. This finding was similar to that reported by McConnell et al. (2002) in their study of the prevalence of psychiatric disorders and care needs in the District of Derry. McConnell et al., who had used the longer GHQ-28 instrument, had detected similar or higher rates of psychiatric disorder in Derry/Londonderry to that found in inner city London, which those researchers concluded were linked to levels of deprivation.

Cairns et al. asked respondents the degree to which they had experienced the Troubles directly or indirectly, and, to what degree they regarded themselves as a victim of the Troubles. Whereas 17% said they had been affected by the Troubles (i.e. high levels of direct or indirect impact), only 12% regarded themselves as 'victims' of the Troubles (i.e. 'often' or 'very often'). The researchers conjectured that this perception by individuals in Northern Ireland – that is, a lower sense of being a victim in relation to experience of the violence – may well be linked to the idea that the Troubles became a way of life or the norm for many people, as reported by the Cost of the Troubles Study (see Chapter 4).

Thinking of oneself as a victim, or as having been impacted upon by the Troubles, were associated with poorer levels of current psychological well-being. The conclusion was that, chiefly, those who had experienced violence directly were carrying the enduring mental health burden linked to the Troubles. With reference to pre-ceasefire studies that used the GHQ (Cairns, 1988; Wilson and Cairns, 1992) and post-ceasefires studies that also used the GHQ (Cairns and Lewis, 1999; Mallet, 2000) the researchers were able to investigate the impact of changing levels of violence. They concluded, 'the ceasefires have not led to any notable change in overall levels of psychological well-being in the Northern Irish population' (Cairns et al., 2003: 2). Whilst being able to determine a relationship between the impact of the Troubles and well-being, the researchers concluded that violence linked to the Troubles is only one of a number of determinants of health.

The psychological impact of the Troubles: 2004

In their review of research, Campbell, Cairns and Mallet (2004) concluded from the work of others they reviewed that the Troubles did not appear to have a major global impact on the mental health of the population. 'Overall, the evidence from these community studies suggests that the majority of people in Northern Ireland were able to cope with low levels of stress associated with political violence. This, of course, is not true for those involved in the most serious incidents, … [and] also for healthcare staff working with the survivors' (p. 179). They concluded that, overall, people had coped through distancing and denial, apart from in circumstances where the violence was so stark that its significance could not be denied. In these circumstances other strategies were deployed. The authors concluded that as a result, the ceasefires have brought little or no psychological benefit because the problems were being coped with. They noted also the interaction between objective and perceived levels of violence, where accurately appraised high levels of violence are associated with poorer mental health.

Key questions arise from the conclusion that there is no major population-wide adverse effect on mental health, and that it is those who experience violence directly who are at greatest risk: what proportion of the population has been exposed to direct experiences of violence and, therefore, how extensive is the risk to and impact upon the well-being of the population? These questions were subsequently addressed in the NICTT-UU series of studies, discussed below.

The legacy of the Troubles: 2005

In 2005, Muldoon et al. reported upon the breadth of conflict experiences in a representative sample of the population in Northern Ireland and the border counties of the Irish Republic. The border counties had been affected by some violence although not with the same level of intensity as in the north. Some people from Northern Ireland had migrated south of the border to the Republic as a result of their experiences of the Troubles. The research team used the GHQ-12 and Post-Traumatic Stress Disorder Checklist – the PCL (Weathers et al., 1993), plus questions to assess drug and alcohol use and dependency, and psychological tough-mindedness. The study relied upon direct questions to ascertain the nature and level of exposure (direct and indirect) to the Troubles. This approach overcame the limitations of relying upon proxy evidence of area-based violence, which may have underestimated the personal experiences of people living in low areas of violence or the effects of migration due to violence or for other reasons.

The study enquired about respondents' experiences (direct and indirect) of the Troubles. Some of the 'experience' types might have involved a trauma or a loss; others (such as being a member of an organisation) might not. Overall, 50% of respondents had no direct experience of the Troubles whereas 20% had three or more experiences. The three most prevalent events were 'experiencing a bomb' (21.5% of men; 18% of women), a riot (26.2% of men; 13.1% of women), and intimidation (25.3% of men; 15% of women).

Those who reported a particularly distressing experience were assessed for PTSD symptoms using the PCL. Overall, 10% met the threshold criteria for PTSD; 12% in the Northern Ireland sample; 6% in the border counties sample. The number and types of event reported were related to the prevalence of PTSD. Participants meeting the PTSD threshold criteria had more Troubles-related experiences (three times for direct and two times for indirect). They were most likely to meet the caseness threshold for PTSD, as a result either of injuries to themselves, incidents that directly affected a friend or family member, or witnessing a killing or violence other than a bombing or shooting. Alcohol and drug use was much greater amongst those who met the criteria for PTSD. On the GHQ-12 the researchers found greater psychological well-being (i.e. lower GHQ scores) than Cairns et al. (2003).

Proposals for a coordinated service trauma network: 2006

At the invitation of Northern Ireland's health department, two people who were both trauma practitioners and service managers prepared a report outlining proposals for a coordinated service network for those suffering psychological and mental health problems arising from the Troubles (Bolton and Healey, 2006).

The authors identified the following challenges in developing therapeutic services in response to the Troubles:

- The level of interest in the victims' issue by political structures is [dependent upon the development of services being] a political necessity i.e. making it to the political agenda.

- To the extent that politics [has addressed] the victims' issue, it is primarily seen as a political issue and not a service or even a reconciliation or peace-building issue.
- The [problem of the] considerable difficulties politicians have in discussing and reaching agreement upon victims' issues (including remembrance and justice) in the context of civil conflict and at times widely different perspectives on the legitimacy of specific categories of victims.
- The need for political consensus on policy, which at times inhibits progressive responses and service developments.
- The difficulties and perhaps impossibility in recognising victims of the Troubles as a special subset of those with service needs (with special provision for accessing services etc.) in the context of equality and targeting social need policies.
- The on-going challenge of embedding Troubles related victims' strategy into existing structures, policies, priorities and commissioning, and provider arrangements.
- The competing positions, arguments and demands of the various services set up to address the consequences of violence or to represent victims.
- In relation to some service areas, the absence of a clear evidence-base, which would inform, legitimise and shape service provision, and upon which strategy and policy could be based.
- Problems created by the way government responsibilities are organised including the split of responsibilities between [regional and national governmental departments], and the difficulties in addressing what was often viewed as a political issue (i.e. the impact of the violence) within mainstream departmental operations. (pp. 2–3)

These realities had inhibited the evolution of strategy and policy 'because predominantly, movement and progress were linked to political necessity [and] what was politically achievable' (p. 3). The authors made a number of policy and service development recommendations. They concluded that a trauma-focused service network focused on service users should be developed to:

- improve information for the public and people likely to come into contact with members of the public who are exposed to and adversely affected by traumatic events;
- achieve the earliest identification of trauma-related needs;
- deliver the most appropriate early responses;
- facilitate speedy referrals to the relevant and identified services (within and beyond a trauma network);
- enable treatments to be provided where possible through [publicly provided] mental health teams and related [not-for-profit] organisations;

- provide access to specialist treatment for chronic and complex trauma-related disorders;
- ensure that service users would have psycho-social support in advance of, during and after treatments. (p. 6)

The authors concluded with a set of service and practice principles, and with a five-year vision for a service based on their proposals.

The effectiveness of the not-for-profit sector: 2007

An investigation by Dillenburger et al. (2007a) of the effectiveness of not-for-profit sector services was undertaken using standardised measures. The researchers assessed 75 adult service users who had been referred to not-for-profit organisations providing counselling and related services for people affected by the Troubles, over a nine to twelve month period. They used the GHQ-30 (Goldberg et al., 1996) and the PDS (Foa et al., 1997). They also used the Personal Experience and Impact of the Troubles Questionnaire (Dillenburger et al., 2007b), the BDI (Beck et al., 1988), and a modified and shortened version of the Stressful Life Events Scale (or Social Re-adjustment Rating Scale) (Holmes and Rahe, 1967) to assess concurrent life stresses.

At the baseline assessment, moderate to high levels of impairment were found; 60% met the caseness threshold on the GHQ-30 (i.e. scoring 5 or more), mean 10.26. The same percentage scored greater than 21 on the PDS (i.e. they met the criteria for moderate to severe PTSD, mean 25.44); 45% scored greater than 19 on the BDI-II, meaning they met the criteria for moderate to severe depressed states, mean 19.32. 'Those who were physically injured or disabled, witnessed a violent incident or were intimidated scored particularly highly when compared with those who did not experience these events' (Dillenburger et al., 2007a; 1638).

Over the twelve or so months of the study, the researchers found improvements in general psychological health and levels of depression associated with services provided by not-for-profit sector services, although the severity of PTSD symptoms did not decrease during the research period. The authors offer a number of explanations including that 'it is possible that the PTSD concept cannot be appropriately applied to individuals who were traumatized by events that happened many years ago' and that traumatic events were still happening during the research period (p. 1643). They emphasised the need to recognise the consequences other stressful life events might have for participants, especially in relation to trauma symptoms. They speculated that those taking part in the study had become chronically traumatised due to the lack of appropriate support at the time of the original traumatic experiences, and therefore would need more specialist interventions. Other reasons offered include the possibility that the study was undertaken at a time of political instability when some violence had been continuing, or because of a lack of justice and recognition. The significant fallout of participants over the study (T1=75; T2=25; T3=20; T4=13) showed something of the problems of carrying out longitudinal studies with groups of service users in a dynamic, uncertain and, at times, violent context where apart from events associated with the conflict, the everyday events in the lives of individuals can disrupt researchers' plans.

The Bamford Review: 2007

In 2007 a major examination of the needs and service requirements of people with mental health and learning disabilities was published (DHSSPS, 2007). The report, which had taken almost ten years to complete, was sponsored by Northern Ireland's health department. It provided a detailed description of the wider mental health (and learning disability) issues in Northern Ireland, setting out the case and ambition for improved services.

In relation to mental health services for adults and communities affected by traumatic experiences, including the Troubles, the report said that, 'The development to date of services has been piecemeal and patchy, and lacks both a managerial and professional coherence' (p. 117). It noted the various adverse mental health and related reactions and needs individuals might have following traumatic experiences, and drew attention to the avoidance-related symptoms of post-trauma reactions that suppress help-seeking. It went on to recommend how trauma services should develop to meet the identified needs of the population, in relation to both conflict and non-conflict trauma stressors. This included a recommendation for a managed service network that would provide service pathways for people suffering trauma-related problems, and link the various components of a comprehensive and integrated service for people exposed to and adversely affected by traumatic events. This would support the early detection, referral, assessment and, if required, therapeutic services for individuals. It would also integrate the contributions of public and not-for-profit service providers, and those non-therapeutic services necessary for the wider support for individuals affected by traumatic events. Regarding standards for trauma treatment services, the review pointed to both the health department's own standards (DHSSPS, 2003) and that published by The National Institute for Clinical Excellence in England and Wales (NICE, 2005). Given the availability of research, guidance and service standards regarding trauma and trauma services the report said there was an opportunity for making progress in the development of trauma-related services.

The report made a number of observations and recommendations regarding the staffing of trauma services. It suggested that staff should be appropriately trained and drawn from a range of professional backgrounds to provide added value and perspective to the assessment and treatment of people with trauma. It recognised the need for different levels of care (i.e. stepped-care) to meet the needs of people with different levels of need, and that staff numbers, experience and the interdisciplinary mix should be appropriate for each level. Service providers should be clear about what they can do and cannot do, and these aims should inform staff recruitment and training.

With reference to the views and needs of potential and current service users, the report included a set of service principles:

- Clear and non-bureaucratic points of access to information and services.
- Proactive awareness of and sensitivity to potential trauma-related needs by key first-point-of-contact professionals and organisations.
- Effective first line responses offering reassurance, clear information, initial care, and onward referral.
- Active response and follow-up to reduce the potential for drop-out associated with avoidance.
- Individualised care to reflect the highly individualistic presentations of trauma-related needs, and the personal associated circumstances (e.g. other illnesses, financial hardships, disability) and any [co-occurring] mental ill-health needs.
- Access to a range of evidence-based therapeutic resources.
- Services should place a clear emphasis on creating a safe and confidential treatment environment.
- Services should have in place key links and arrangements to respond to urgent and other needs that cannot be met within the specific service. (DHSSPS, 2007: 118)

The report contained a number of recommendations relating to the development of trauma-related services, including recommendations on service development plans, training and community education.

Evaluation of therapy for PTSD sufferers: 2007

Duffy et al. (2007) undertook a randomised controlled trial of trauma-focused cognitive behavioural therapy (CBT) for adults suffering PTSD and other disorders linked to the Troubles. The study detailed patients' experiences, the complexity of needs arising from these, and subsequent trauma-related mental health problems, yielding important insights into the impact of multiple traumatic experiences, latency (i.e. delayed on-set of trauma-related symptoms) and help-seeking. The findings showed that patients with multiple trauma exposure and severe PTSD made significant progress with trauma-focused CBT compared to those on a waiting list. This was one of the studies undertaken by the Northern

Ireland Centre for Trauma and Transformation (NICTT) and is discussed further in Chapter 9.

Social identification and trauma in Northern Ireland: 2007

Following up on Muldoon et al. (2005), Muldoon and Downes (2007) reported on an investigation of exposure to the Troubles, trauma symptoms, identity and demographic characteristics. The study, undertaken in 2004, involved a sample of 3,000 telephone interviewees comparable to the general population of Northern Ireland and the border counties of the Republic of Ireland: 42% reported a distressing event linked to the Troubles. (This is comparable to the 39% of adults who had at least one traumatic experience linked to the conflict found by the NICTT-UU research partnership – see below.) This group was then assessed for PTSD symptoms using the PCL (Weathers et al., 1993): 10% of respondents met the criteria for PTSD, with double the prevalence of PTSD in Northern Ireland (12%) compared with the Republic of Ireland (6%). The group meeting PTSD criteria reported over twice the number of direct, and almost twice the number of indirect, Troubles-related distressing events. The PTSD group also attributed lower levels of importance to national identity, was more likely to have lower educational attainment, lower mean incomes, and be less likely to be in employment. Importantly, the PTSD group were much more likely than the total sample to consider themselves to be victims of the Troubles, although within this group 46% never or rarely considered themselves as such (p. 149). Muldoon and Downes conclude that this 'non-victim' PTSD group could miss out on policies and services promoted as being for victims of the Troubles. (See Cairns et al., 2003; Bunting et al., 2012.) Their findings suggest that trauma exposure and the subsequent development of trauma-related disorders should be considered in policy, service and practice terms mindful of previous and multiple traumatic experiences, adverse socio-economic circumstances, and the absence or loss of group solidarity.

This study added to the consideration of how perceptions and identity interact with traumatic experiences and deprivation in the context of conflict. The authors surmise that a strong social or national identity might be protective in the face of traumatic experiences, with implications for post-conflict policies and service design and delivery.

The Interim Victims Commissioner's Report: 2007

In her report to government, the Interim Victims Commissioner reviewed the provision of services for those affected by the Troubles (McDougal, 2007). She noted areas of unmet need, such as those bereaved and injured in the early years of the conflict, and those suffering chronic pain. The Commissioner acknowledged the efforts of services to respond to the needs of those affected by violence. In spite of the need she concluded there was 'no evidence of an acknowledgement in the [publicly provided] sector that there is a need to raise awareness of victims' and survivors' issues' and that 'the service delivery model is too complex, is not easily understood and does not appear to be working' (p. iv). She concluded that service developments (including those relating to mental health and trauma) had been patchy and uncoordinated and recommended that services should be brought under the responsibility of the publicly provided health and social care system and developed in line with the Bamford Report (DHSSPS, 2007). She noted that people with needs relating to the Troubles had problems in getting them recognised and responded to effectively, and recommended that training for family doctors should be provided to assist in the screening for PTSD. She also recommended that counselling services for those affected by the Troubles should be accredited to recognised standards.

The Commissioner reported that over £44 million of central government and European Union funding had been spent on those affected by the Troubles. This included £36.4 million allocated by central government since 1998 and £12.7 million from the European Union's Peace programmes for Northern Ireland and the border counties of the Republic of Ireland (p. v).

The NICTT-UU series of epidemiological studies: 2008–2014

Between 2008 and 2012 a partnership of the NICTT and the Psychology Research Institute at Ulster University (UU) published a series of studies that examined the mental and associated physical health impact of the Troubles. The NICTT-UU partnership drew upon primary data from the Northern Ireland Study of Health and Stress (NISHS), one of thirty or so identical studies undertaken across the world under the auspices of the World Mental Health Survey Initiative (Kessler et al., 2009). The research team found that adults' levels of exposure to conflict and non-conflict-related traumatic events (60.6%) were slightly below international norms of around two thirds for developed societies (Galea et al., 2005). Nearly four in ten adults (39%) had been exposed to one or more conflict-related traumatic events (see, Muldoon et al., 2005; and Muldoon and Downes, 2007). The level of twelve-month PTSD (conflict and non-conflict-related) was estimated to be 5.1%; the lifetime level was 8.8%. The conditional level (i.e. the proportion of those who, having been exposed to traumatic events, subsequently met the criteria for PTSD) was 15% (compared to Muldoon et al.'s (2005) finding of 12%). Conflict-related traumatic events were associated with much higher levels of PTSD. This pattern was observed across a wide range of mental health disorders. Exposure to conflict-related traumatic events was found to be a marker for higher levels of mental ill-health and was associated with deprivation and other determinants of adverse health and well-being. The partnership investigated help-seeking and found that those meeting the criteria for anxiety disorders, which includes PTSD, take on average twenty-two years to seek help (Ferry et al., 2008; Bunting et al., 2012) The series also included an assessment of the health-related economic costs of PTSD in Northern Ireland (Ferry et al., 2011). The studies are discussed further in Chapter 9.

The Troubles in north and west Belfast: 2008

A report by Dorahy et al. (2008) summarised three important studies undertaken by practitioners from the Trauma Resource Centre, a publicly funded centre delivering services to the local population in north and west Belfast. This area experienced some of the greatest intensity of violence linked to the Troubles. The local population experienced 'sectarian attacks, attacks on security forces and state violence [with] … neighbourhoods being regulated and policed by their own paramilitary group members' (p. 6). The population also suffered higher than average social deprivation, high unemployment, and cultural and community division. Even following the ceasefires of the early and mid-1990s, the area continued to experience violence linked to circumstances and groups associated with the conflict. The first study examined the level of exposure to the Troubles in childhood and adulthood of three service user groups. One group comprised patients attending the centre. The second was a sample drawn from patients attending a rural adult psychology department, and the third, patients from a hospital-based programme for people with severe and enduring mental illness. Using The Troubles-Related Experiences Questionnaire (Dorahy, Shannon and Maguire, 2007) the researchers found that the levels of both childhood and adult exposure to the Troubles, and the assessed objective and subjective impact on the life of the person, were substantially and significantly higher amongst those attending the centre compared to the other samples. These findings endorsed earlier conclusions by Fay et al. (1998) that the population of north and west Belfast had suffered significant levels of exposure to Troubles-related traumatic events. This high level of exposure to conflict-related violence, coupled with high levels of social and economic deprivation, and adverse childhood experiences, accounted for the high levels and complexity of psychological and mental health related problems amongst those attending the centre.

The Consultative Group on the Past: 2009

Under the joint leadership of two well-known public figures from Northern Ireland, Lord Robin Eames and Denis Bradley, the Consultative Group was established in 2007 by the British Secretary of State 'to find a way forward out of the shadows of the past … to enable our society to do this together, to be achieved through the widest possible consultation' (Eames et al., 2009: 14).

On the basis of extensive consultations, the Group wove together a detailed commentary, balancing many differing and often opposing views, and brought forward a series of integrated recommendations that they believed would, on the basis of their consultations, create the means to effectively, yet safely and constructively, deal with the past – that is, those issues from the years of conflict and violence that remained unresolved, and that threaten or impede peace and political progress. In relation to mental health they concluded that:

> Conflict-related trauma is a major public health issue. More than many other issues it has the capacity to pass on a negative legacy to future generations. … The provision of mental health services needs to take fuller account of the mental health legacy of the conflict and reflect this in both the provision of services and ongoing operational priorities. (p. 88)

In relation to the understanding of, and responses to trauma, the Group concluded that 'more needs to be done to create a greater understanding of trauma, to ensure effective responses to it, adequate service provision and the accessibility of those services' (p. 30).

The Group noted the problems and gaps in service accessibility. They observed that there were different views held by 'many dedicated people working in this very complex area' (p. 88) on the best way forward, and recommended that better mechanisms be developed to ensure people get the help they need at the right time for them, noting that 'during the conflict people did not always have the time, understanding, or support to deal with their symptoms and pain' (p. 88).

Public services were regarded by some who met the Group as 'inflexible and unduly wedded to certain therapeutic responses, some of which may not be the most effective' (p. 88). Underlying funding problems needed long-term and strategic solutions. Carers of victims and survivors had unmet needs. The Group also registered the call for comparable levels of services for civilians, as for those provided for the police and army.

Under one of the recommended structures they advised that a range of matters should be addressed, including sectarianism, remembering activities, the needs of and risks to young people (to ensure there is no repeat of the past), equality in the economic benefits for deprived areas, and the enabling of those exiled from Northern Ireland during the conflict to return home. In relation to mental health, the Group wished to see 'improved services to meet healthcare needs attributable to the conflict, including dealing with trauma, suicide and addiction issues (p. 38).

Strategy for Victims and Survivors: 2009

This strategy, published by the central department of the Northern Ireland Government, provided a framework for future policy and services. It described an architecture comprising a Commission for Victims and Survivors, a Victims and Survivors Forum and a Victims and Survivors Service. The document also contained aims for the new policy and a set of principles (OFMDFM, 2009). In terms of needs the document noted:

> What is important varies greatly from individual to individual. Many face the consequences of trauma and/or physical disability. There remains a demand for support services including counselling, befriending and a variety of therapies while for many people simply getting information about available services is a problem.
>
> Some victims and survivors wish to find out more about the circumstances surrounding the death of a relative. Many suffer financial hardship, social isolation, exclusion and a variety of problems arising from loss or injury. There are those who wish to have their individual stories heard, documented, archived, shared and appropriately acknowledged. Public acknowledgement including memorials and other forms of public recognition is also important to many people. (p. 3).

Guidance from Northern Ireland's health department: 2010–2011

In a consultation paper from Northern Ireland's health department, views were sought on a future strategy for social work. It observed that, 'many people in Northern Ireland remain affected by bereavement, trauma, violence and the challenge of adjusting to life in a post-conflict society' (DHSSPS, 2010: 5). In the following year, the health department's Service Framework for Mental Health and Wellbeing noted that:

> Northern Ireland has a higher overall prevalence of mental health problems; that is 25% higher than in England. Northern Ireland has a unique range of problems as a result of … 'the troubles'. There is a high level of socio-economic deprivation, which is worse in some geographical areas by the prolonged effect of 'the troubles'. Within the population there remains a great deal of hurt, anger, sadness and trauma problems that have affected the mental health and wellbeing of people in (Northern Ireland). (DHSSPS, 2011: 59)

In a detailed overview of PTSD and the risks of co-occurring disorders and needs, the Service Framework included specific recommendations derived from best practice guidance as to how people with PTSD, including those affected by conflict-related events, should be treated by the public mental health services. It advised that:

> A person with a confirmed diagnosis of post traumatic stress disorder should have access to timely psychological and social interventions, medication and treatment

appropriate to their needs, delivered by suitably qualified and supervised practitioners. A standardised outcome measurement tool should be used in treatment and care. (p. 186)

Heenan and Birrell: 2011

In a wide-ranging review of the contribution and experiences of social workers and the discipline of social work in relation to the Troubles, Heenan and Birrell (2011) observed a developing focus on trauma-related mental health needs. They considered two studies which examined the views of social workers in relation to the Troubles (Smyth et al. 2001; Campbell and McCrystal, 2005). Focusing on the implications of violence for social work they identified five distinct effects. These were, that the Troubles had:

1. created special and unique needs;
2. added a unique context to 'normal' social work services;
3. given rise to special obstacles to delivering services;
4. placed pressures on some staff workloads, and
5. generated adverse stress, trauma-related risks and consequences. (adapted from Heenan and Birrell, 2011: 38)

Drawing upon research and public service documents, the authors tracked the developments in relation to the mental health and related impacts on individuals and communities, considered the impact of violence on the social work staff of service providers, and reviewed the contribution of social work to disaster management. They noted that it was in 1995 (see DHSS, 1998) that Northern Ireland's health department launched a project to 'develop services to meet the social and psychological needs of individuals affected by the conflict', which included the creation of crisis response teams in parts of Northern Ireland whose aims were to provide immediate and structured responses 'to those affected by terrorist-related incidents' (p. 45).

The needs of those injured as a result of the Troubles: 2012

Breen-Smyth (2012) undertook a study for WAVE, a regional victims and survivors organisation working in Northern Ireland, with funding from the Office of the First Minister and Deputy First Minister, the central department of Northern Ireland's Government. An overarching objective was to address the lack of recognition, attention to and knowledge of the consequences of the Troubles for those who were injured, with a particular focus on those who were disabled as a consequence, plus their families and carers. The study investigated physical injury, defined for the purposes of the study as 'life threatening or disfiguring physical injury'. Psychological injury was also assessed in relation to those meeting the definition of physical injury.

The researcher identified two key areas that had a bearing on general functioning. The first was the need to manage complex medical needs. This included dependence on others and public health services, mobility limitations, increased personal safety needs, adverse impacts on work, family and relationships and other daily living problems. The second area with implications for general functioning was the consequences for the psychological state of injured and disabled persons. This included a range of disorders, chiefly mood and anxiety disorders; the use of, dependence upon or misuse of prescribed medication, illegal drugs and alcohol; adverse impacts upon social functioning and on the person's sense of purpose; social isolation; and feelings of anger.

The report made a considerable number of recommendations in relation to:

- financial support for injured people and their families;
- welfare, mental health and well-being;
- justice;
- integration;
- victims' policy, service development and acknowledgement, and
- further research to determine the size of the injured population.

In relation to mental health specifically, the study used the PDS (Foa et al., 1997) to assess the level of PTSD in a survey of seventy-six injured adults, which sixty-five (85.5%) completed. Respondents were assessed in terms of PDS four severity categories. Less than 4% of the sample (three respondents) scored at the mild end of the scale; 6.6% (five respondents) scored as 'moderate'; 75% (fifty-seven respondents) scored as either 'moderate to severe' or 'severe' on the PDS scale. The 'moderate to severe' group comprised 87% of the respondents who completed the PDS scale.

The CVSNI Comprehensive Needs Assessment: 2012

The Commission for Victims and Survivors for Northern Ireland (CVSNI) was established in 2008, following the passing of legislation by the Northern Ireland Assembly in 2006 (Victims and Survivors (Northern Ireland) Order 2006). The development of a comprehensive needs-assessment was a core objective of the Commission so that it could advise Northern Ireland's Executive and Assembly and the British Government in London on needs and service requirements. A specific aim of the comprehensive needs-assessment was to provide early advice for the anticipated Victims and Survivors Service due to be established in 2012. The Commission published its Comprehensive Needs Assessment in 2012 (CVSNI, 2012). In concluding its analysis of the needs of those affected by the years of conflict, the Commission identified the following priorities as the basis of its advice to government, commencing with the most pressing concerns.

- Health and Wellbeing.
- Social Support.
- Individual Financial Needs.
- Truth, Justice and Acknowledgement.
- Welfare Support.
- Trans-generational Issues and Young People.
- Personal and Professional Development.

With a view to informing the development and work of the planned Victims and Survivors Service, the Commission made a series of recommendations. In relation to mental health, these were informed by the Troubled Consequences Report (Bunting et al., 2012) that had been funded by the Commission. (This was a compilation and extension of some of the NICTT-UU series of studies discussed above.)

The Commission encouraged consideration of developing a trauma-focused coordinated service network (based on the model of a managed clinical network) by key governmental departments in Northern Ireland that would 'deliver a comprehensive regional trauma service drawing largely on existing resources and expertise from the statutory [publicly provided] independent and voluntary [not-for-profit] sectors' (pp. 13 & 44). The Commission concluded that given the amount of health-related needs, the planned Victims and Survivors Service would need to 'ensure there is sufficient capacity to address the assessed mental and physical health needs of victims and survivors in a timely and effective manner' (p. 12). To achieve this the Commission recommended that the Service undertake a capacity building exercise and prepare workforce development plans 'to ensure appropriately qualified practitioners are available at each level of intervention' (p. 12). Also in the light of the evidence of mental health related need that the 'service should consider developing a general mental healthcare pathway to effectively capture and treat these and other mental health disorders' (p. 12). This would require a package of 'intensive interventions' guided by evidence-based practice such as that described in the guidance issued by the National Institute for Health and Care Excellence (NICE, 2005) and DHSSPS (2003). These developments should be guided by key themes including a focus on recovery, a stepped-care approach to mental health and a holistic assessment model that assesses underlying mental and physical health conditions. In view of the specific problem of late help-seeking, the Commission urged progress in early detection and help-seeking particularly among individuals with anxiety and alcohol or drugs related disorders.

Shoulder to Shoulder: Moving Forward: 2013

In 2013 the Sandy Row Community Forum published a report which had been commissioned to investigate the context of emotional well-being for the community of ex-combatants (i.e. former armed group activists) from the Protestant-Unionist-Loyalist community in south Belfast, and to assess the approach to emotional health and well-being needs for that community (Sandy Row Community Forum, 2013). The study was funded by Northern Ireland's Public Health Agency and relied upon peer researchers from the community to engage with, and gather data from, participants. The study identified social and economic factors in the neighbourhoods in which the ex-combatants were living that were impacting upon health. In relation to the ex-combatants themselves, 'The study identified particular concerns about the emotional and mental health of the respondents, particularly in regard to disconnection, isolation with feelings of abandonment that has resulted in high levels of depression and expressed suicidal thoughts' (p. 7). Respondents felt that their past experiences had impacted more significantly on their psychological health than their physical health, with evidence of depression and suicidal thoughts. The researchers found high levels of alcohol use and evidence of the on-going psychological impact of historic traumatic events. Many respondents felt shunned and isolated within their community because of their former roles and activities, with implications for integration and access to services. Changes in community perceptions, which no longer saw them as positive figures but ones that should be avoided, were impacting upon their social contact and feelings of well-being, with concerns about being alone in their old age. They felt unable to talk frankly with others who might be able to help them, due to concerns about how their former activities might be judged and because of anxieties about continuing or new investigations into past events.

The researchers drew attention to the distinctive and worrying levels of poor psychological health and well-being of this group of respondents. The report highlights the problems faced by a group of actors in conflict who, when the violence ends, face considerable problems in re-framing their past roles and aims in the new political context, and who have to contend with major shifts in how they are perceived within their own community. The problems give rise to difficulties in reintegrating (e.g. being accepted, getting work) and in getting access to services that are capable of handling the unique circumstances of their past, and their psychological, physical and other health-related needs. Concern for those who may have been responsible for violence, as noted earlier, comes into conflict with the views and expectations of many who have been the subjects of that violence, posing major issues for a post-conflict community and its politics.

Evidence of the intergenerational impact of the Troubles: 2015

The intergenerational impact of adverse experiences is an established theme in various areas of research, practice and service delivery. Previous researchers, including many of those included in this review, signalled various levels of concern or raised questions as to the longer-term consequences of the years of violence on subsequent generations. In Northern Ireland, practitioners and service providers working with communities and families in mental health and in education, the criminal justice sector, and in areas or with groups adversely affected by the Troubles had been aware of consequential effects of the civil discord on subsequent generations, although the nature and scale of the problem lacked definition. Various reports had identified this as a distinct concern. For example, the 2009 Consultative Group on the Past (see above) had, on the basis of extensive consultations, observed that:

> Inter-generational trauma is similarly not recognised as a root cause of the problems many young people face. Many are affected by the legacy of the past while often having only indirect experience of that past. (Eames et al., 2009: 87)

Another report from the Irish Peace Centres on the basis of an extensive review of the international literature on the trans-generational impacts of conflict and focus groups in Ireland concluded:

> that the intergenerational transmission of the experience of conflict in Northern Ireland corresponds with international trends identified in the research literature. Namely, that the effects of harm (broadly defined) and the experience of injustice carried by a particular generation can, if not addressed or resolved, be passed on to the next generation to produce a range of social and psychological pathologies, such as self- harm, suicide, anti-social behaviour, anomie and inter-personal violence. (Irish Peace Centres, 2010: 78)

In 2012 The Commission for Victims and Survivors published research it had commissioned into this area. The researchers identified the need for more research on this matter in Northern Ireland, given the 'dearth of research specifically examining trans-generational trauma in the specific context of the Troubles' (Hanna et al., 2012: 6). On the basis of a study involving a small sample of participants, the researchers identified how survivors had normalised violence as an expected part of life, which may have led to seeing the world as an unsafe place and therefore resulted in hyper-protection of their children. This led to shielding of children from the Troubles, including reluctance to discuss the violence, and a lack of disclosure about personal experiences of (or involvement in) violence. The researchers found some evidence that transmissions of trauma from parents who experienced violence to their children may have contributed to anxiety, hyper-vigilance and depression. They identified therapy and opportunities to share experiences of the Troubles as possible means of helping.

Working with families and uncovering underlying traumatic experiences within families were identified by therapists as key methods in working with families affected by trans-generational trauma. A survey of young people undertaken by the researchers,

> provided evidence that trans-generational trauma is a very real issue in Northern Ireland … with (most) respondents reporting that they had experienced trauma-related events, but also … that their family's experiences of the Troubles have had a greater impact on them than their own experience. (Hanna et al., 2012: 8)

The Commission subsequently funded further research to take forward the work of Hanna et al. Comprising a series of papers and an overview of the main conclusions and recommendations, this second report into the trans-generational consequences of the Troubles examined the issue from a number of perspectives (O'Neill et al., 2015). Through literature and research reviews, secondary analysis of data from earlier research and surveys of service providers working in the public and not-for-profit sectors, the research team's approach was to better understand the possible range of adverse outcomes for children and adults arising from personal or parental exposure to violence associated with the Troubles and to assess current service availability.

The researchers concluded that whilst most people in Northern Ireland have not suffered long-term problems linked to the Troubles, about 15% of adults have mental health difficulties that appear to be associated with the civil violence. They concluded that adverse experiences of conflict-related violence, consequential mental health problems, and other socio-economic disadvantages and stressors on adults, impact on the parenting of their children. Harsh, neglectful and otherwise poor parenting styles, especially where worsened by economic and social stressors, impact on the developing child – limiting the development of attachments, emotional competence (self-regulation), social skills and other capabilities. These then place the child at increased risks of a range of disadvantages in childhood, adolescence and later in adulthood – including poorer mental health, which is made worse by poverty and other basic deprivations. In turn, this secondary wave of adversity and disadvantage is more likely to impact negatively on the next generation, and so on.

In the context of societal conflict, this sequence of disadvantage can also be the means through which unresolved narratives of the conflict, laden with fearful, aggressive or sectarian sentiments, are conveyed across generations. This cyclical transmission of adverse experiences and their consequences can, if it reaches a critical mass in a community, contribute to new episodes of organised violence (Maedl et al., 2010). Not surprisingly, one of the key themes of the report was the merit of addressing the developing post-conflict pattern of need on an intergenerational basis, to include systemic or family focused interventions, for example.

Two of the research team undertook a secondary analysis of data from the Northern Ireland Study of Heath and Stress (NISHS – the data-set used by the NICTT-UU research partnership discussed above), examining the associations and causal relationships amongst harsh or maltreatment experiences in childhood, exposure to conflict-related traumatic experiences and mental illness, including suicidal behaviours (McKenna and Bunting, 2015). The researchers concluded that 'respondents whose parents suffered from mental illness and who engage in physically aggressive parenting practices were more likely to have been exposed to conflict-related (traumas)' (p. 66). The offspring of these parents are vulnerable to the same risks of childhood toxic stress that they themselves were exposed to, if for different reasons. Pointing to the mechanisms of intergenerational transmission of adversity, they also concluded that, 'the children of these subgroups may be particularly vulnerable in terms of trauma transmission' (p. 67). To break the cycle of intergenerational poverty, trauma transmission and prejudice transmission, the authors recommended programmes that would promote parents' capacities to manage their households and secure employment. This included investment in parents with trauma-related mental health disorders to help them overcome the consequences of both their childhood and conflict traumas.

In the same report, through a survey of organisations working with neighbourhoods or more widely, and with groups that had experienced the Troubles, respondents were invited to indicate their views on the intergenerational consequences and priorities (Bolton and Devine, 2015). The findings point to mental ill health, substance abuse and addiction as the foremost health-related problems. These were followed by a range of interpersonal and family difficulties, then by problems that were associated with missed opportunities in educational attainment, personal development and development of self-esteem. These priorities came ahead of the truth and justice related concerns associated with the Troubles – that arose out of desire for truth about what happened to loved ones, for example, or justice for those who were killed, injured or otherwise adversely affected. These might have been expected to loom larger in a community affected by civil conflict. Parents were regarded as requiring the most support in relation to their own needs and in supporting their parenting function within families. The findings were broadly endorsed by the views of mental health and therapy service managers and practitioners in both the public and not-for-profit sectors.

The implication is that, as communities move away from conflict-related violence, the consequences of the direct experiences of violence recede and are increasingly replaced by the more diffuse everyday concerns and problems of deprived or stressed individuals, families and neighbourhoods – which to one degree or another have their origins in experiences of conflict-related violence. The risks are that damaging experiences of violence give rise to adverse parenting styles, which impact on the next generation in developmental terms. This in turn places the child, adolescent and emerging adult at a disadvantage across various areas – including mental health. This can contribute to new occasions for cynicism over being left behind as politics progresses, with associated grievance and resentment, and potentially leave disaffected individuals open to embracing violence. This process creates vectors for the transmission of narratives and group sentiments that perpetuate, or give rise to new episodes of, violence. To address this complex pattern of need, policy and service responses are required to address the enduring and now chronic needs of those who have directly experienced the violence of the Troubles, and also the emerging complex needs arising from developmental and economic deprivations, and the changing nature of violence in a post-conflict setting. Whilst all age ranges could benefit from support and additional services, parents – as the pivot between the past and the future, as those who witnessed and endured the violence and yet have to bring up a new generation – are key.

Wider policies and interventions are required that address problems at national or community levels, for example, social measures that address poverty and broad parenting challenges and deficits. Narrower actions are likewise needed at the family and personal levels, to address the skills needs, psychological and mental health disorders, developmental, and inter-generational needs, of individuals and families.

Suicide trends: findings from later studies

Many of the studies discussed above address the issue of suicide. Three later papers are considered here. In a detailed consideration of suicide trends in Northern Ireland, since the early days of the Troubles up until well after the Belfast Agreement, Tomlinson (2007, 2012 and 2013) noted the relatively low levels of suicide-related deaths in the earlier years, but cautioned against the reliability of this early data in view of practical and stigma-related problems in the processing and recording of deaths. He noted the marked increase in suicide-related deaths following the Belfast Agreement. He offered a number of observations, including the adverse social and economic impact of war and civil conflict on opportunities, integration and segregation. His main finding was that the highest rates of suicide appear to be amongst those who experienced the worst period of the Troubles. This part of the population, which had been 'the most acculturated to division and conflict, and to externalized expressions of aggression' (Tomlinson, 2013: 8) now found that, as a result of peace, 'such expressions of aggression and violence are no longer socially approved. They become internalized instead' (p. 8).

In a secondary analysis of data from the NISHS, O'Neill et al. (2014) assessed the associations of conflict-related and non-conflict-related traumatic events with suicidal behaviour. (See also the NICTT-UU series of epidemiological studies

(2008–2014), above.) Respondents were assigned to one of three sub categories: (1) those who had never had a traumatic experience; (2) those who had had only one or more non-conflict-related traumatic experiences; and (3) those who had had one or more conflict-related traumatic experience. The methodology controlled for age, gender and the effects of mental health disorders. Although suicidal ideation and attempts were more common in women than men, rates of suicide plans were similar for both genders. People with mood, anxiety and substance disorders were significantly more likely than those without to have thought about suicide, made plans or made an attempt.

The probability of seriously considering suicide was significantly higher for people with conflict-related and non-conflict-related traumatic experiences compared with people who had never experienced a traumatic event. However, suicide attempts were significantly higher for people who had had only non-conflict-related traumatic experiences compared with the other two categories. The researchers concluded that these findings might be explained by a higher rate of single, fatal suicide attempts among people who have had one or more conflict-related traumatic experiences.

O'Neill (2015) considered the association between the Troubles and suicide thinking, planning and attempts. She offered a number of possible explanations for the numbers of suicides, which at the time, were rising in Northern Ireland. Over the course of the Troubles, the population of Northern Ireland had a high level of exposure to conflict-related violence and associated traumatic events (Bunting et al., 2013). O'Neill notes the contribution of exposure to or involvement in traumatic events and violence to the acquisition of a capability for suicide (Klonsky and May, 2014). Based upon the analysis of data from the NISHS, the predictors of suicidal thinking, planning and attempts point to an association between exposure to traumatic events and suicidal behaviours.

Mental health disorders are predictive of suicidal behaviours, and the higher levels in the NISHS of more serious mental health disorders associated with conflict-trauma exposure were found to be associated with higher levels of suicidal behaviour (Bunting et al., 2013; Ferry et al., 2014). Also in the NISHS, those who had had one or more traumatic experiences, and in particular traumatic experiences linked to conflict, were much more likely to have one or more mental health disorders. Exposure to conflict-related traumatic experiences was also associated with impulse control symptoms and disorders and with higher levels of alcohol and drug misuse and dependency. Both these were associated with suicidal behaviours. O'Neill concludes that whilst it is difficult to provide accurate estimates of the proportions, 'it is reasonable to suggest that many of the suicides associated with those mental disorders are also therefore a consequence of (conflict-related) traumatic events' (O'Neill, 2015: 72).

Discussion

Since the Troubles erupted in 1969, as the above overview illustrates, many researchers have sought to explore whether, to what degree, and in what ways the violence has impacted on the mental health and well-being of individuals and communities. Broadly speaking, the early efforts found little evidence of an adverse impact, contrasting with some of the later studies, which have reported significant if not alarming levels of mental disorders and associated problems, with arresting evidence of the impact on subsequent generations. In the midst of this collection of studies are findings, from Cairns et al. for example, that most people in Northern Ireland seem to have coped with the violence well, managing it by distancing themselves psychologically from the realties and immediacy of the violence. And when the violence is unavoidable, adopting strategies that accepted the realities but contained it through cohesiveness within communities, or by reframing its meaning and threat. One or two studies found evidence of a positive effect from the violence with improved, rather than reduced, psychological well-being.

The studies cover a period of over forty years – embracing the period of the Troubles and the post-political agreement period. In broad terms the Troubles began with a period of protest that quickly led to an explosive eruption of violence, largely street based. This gave way to bombings of political and economic targets, then increased sectarian and other assassinations, followed by a period when culture and rights were fought over in street protests and disputes. Finally the violence entered a period of occasional acts of violence by non-state armed groups and individuals that had not endorsed the peace process and the political settlements of the Belfast and subsequent agreements, with occasional spasms of street protest and violence. Throughout this period the role of different players in the violence changed, with the forces of the state (the army and police mainly) being perceived as protector or enemy, or as holding the line between warring interests, groups and communities. Non-state armed groups were perceived at various times as protectors or oppressors of their own communities, and as a threat to the state or to the other community. In the midst of this extended period of violent conflict, mental health and other services and practitioners endeavoured to address the everyday and violence-linked needs of individuals, families and neighbourhoods. Several reports, considered above, record and acknowledge the commitment of services and practitioners to addressing the needs arising from the Troubles (e.g. McDougal, 2007; Eames et al., 2009; Bolton and Devine, 2014).

It is particularly interesting that much of the substantive evidence for the adverse impact of the Troubles on the population began to emerge just as the process that led to the political settlement of the Belfast Agreement was getting underway. From the research and service delivery evidence, it is clear that the violent contexts of the Troubles, their origins and co-existing social and economic stresses, the fears they generated, the breakdown of trust, the inability to cooperate, the direct, indirect and sometimes multiple experiences of hostility and violence, and their duration over many years, can now be seen collectively as a sustained and formidable social determinant of health and well-being in Northern Ireland's population (Wilkinson, 2011). Further, several authoritative studies have noted that Northern Ireland has comparably greater mental health needs with comparably lower expenditure on services (Appleby, 2005; DHSSPS, 2007; Appleby, 2011). Bengoa et al. (2016) noted the findings of Appleby's studies (2005 and 2011): 'Appleby's review also found … mental health needs in Northern Ireland were estimated to be nearly 44% higher than in England, while actual per capita spending on these services was in fact 10–30% lower.' (p. 34)

Looking at why evidence of the high impact of the Troubles emerged in more recent years invites a number of possibilities and reasons to be considered. One reading might be that the initial drama of the early violence was broadly containable psychologically, held within rationales of civil rights on one hand and defence on the other. Muldoon and Downes's (2007) consideration that strong national and social identities could be protective, might have been particularly relevant during the early years as the political and violent lines were being formed. As the impact intensified, and losses and the traumatic events experienced by individuals, families and communities multiplied, these ideological positions could not hold. Arguably the political realisations in London, Belfast and Dublin, and on the streets and country lanes of Northern Ireland, that the war could not be won by anyone, was a political version of the personal cognitive and emotional realisation that this conflict did not make sense any more. When the peace settlement came, fragile and tentative though it has been, the settlement was out of tune with the psychological infrastructure within which the losses and trauma had been borne. In one way the losses (i.e. the deaths) had been understood in terms of grief, certainly by those families and friends who experienced them. Collectively, the losses were also felt as a tally of the losses of each party to the conflict. Politics was moving on and whilst this was necessary and desired by many, it left in its wake the need for acknowledgement, unresolved injustices and needs that had been endured but which now needed responses. It was in this period that there was an outpouring. After the Belfast Agreement, many self-help groups were formed (Dillenburger et al., 2008; 16), not only to secure services but to say, 'remember us' and 'remember what you did to us'. And it was in this period that the underlying psychological wound of the Troubles started to become more visible. This resonates with the conclusions of writers such as Leed (1979) who viewed the adverse mental health impact of the First World War as a complex psycho-social phenomenon, wherein he discusses the part played by context and meaning on the presentation of war neuroses. He notes Graves and Hodge's (1941) observation that 'those who managed to avoid a nervous breakdown during the war collapsed badly in 1921 or 22' (Leed, 1979: 188).

A further explanation might be found in considering the significance of the ceasefires and their breakdown in the mid-1990s. In 1994 the ceasefires that prefaced the commencement of political talks were in place, with the IRA calling its ceasefire in August, followed by a number of loyalist groups in October. The IRA broke its ceasefire in early 1996. This was reinstated in 1997 (Curtis, 2014). The first IRA ceasefire was widely received with enthusiasm, popularly being regarded as the definitive end of the conflict, even though significant and difficult politics lay ahead. This sentiment was reflected in the extensive and largely unguarded accounts of personal experiences of the years of violence on the broadcast media and in newsprint. There was a sense of 'the lid coming off' and much that had been suppressed and managed up to that point was now being very freely expressed. The breakdown of the IRA ceasefire in 1996 brought this to a grinding halt, and when the ceasefire was reinstated in 1997, the response was more muted and guarded and a degree of collective cynicism entered the public mind.

The difficulties of undertaking research in the context of the Troubles has been noted above, and is further discussed in Chapter 9. The methods and approaches used by researchers also seem to have played their part in the slow discovery of the impact of the violence. Several writers and research teams included in this overview observed that using studies which relied on methods assessing changes in use of services, and changes in the numbers being diagnosed with one or other mental health disorders, was not a reliable approach to investigating the impact of the Troubles. Partly this is because the violence itself changed people's behaviour. Streets blocked by riots or the fear of being caught up in violence acted as a real barrier to service access and help-seeking. Over time, the violence became the new norm. People simply habituated to the daily drip, drip of violence and the relatively low levels of stress it invoked (McWhirter, 1987). They developed new skills: for instance, people were able to judge the degree to which the violence posed a threat to them personally. This was moderated by their sense of their profile as a target, and the sense of danger they perceived them or their family might be in as casual collateral victims And they had developed behavioural and conversational styles that limited their exposure to danger. They had developed skills and confidence in navigating perceived risks in terms of unnecessarily drawing attention to themselves by being careful about what they said and where they said it, or avoiding places, totally or at times, which they might have regarded as being dangerous. Mistrust of services, where fears that personal information and details about one's role in the violence or the response to violence might be inappropriately disclosed, surely played a part. Also, there is evidence from some of the studies that some people might have improved psychologically from the violence and the violent context around them (e.g. Loughrey and Curran, 1987).

Second, Allen et al. (1994) – having examined their own and previous studies of the impact of the Troubles – suggested that the variation in the levels of mental disorders linked to the conflict 'may be due to the changing nature of the violence or the more recent studies may reflect the consequences of longterm exposure to violence' (p. 69). Third, and as noted above, several of the studies demonstrate that it is not enough to ask about service usage. Deloitte and Touche (2003) undertook a literature review and concluded that it 'provided sufficient evidence to question the validity of utilisation based data in certain services and subgroups of the population' (p. 15). They therefore made the case for reference to epidemiological (i.e. population based) data to obtain a more accurate picture of need. Writing in 2008, Murphy concluded that, 'we are still unsure as to the extent of the effects of long-term low-intensity warfare [in Northern Ireland] as no uniform and strategic research on psychological health and well-being has taken place' (Murphy, 2008: 60).

Bell et al. (1988; Kee et al., 1987) found in their audit of 499 people affected by the Troubles that a total of 15.5% required psychiatric services, yet 23% met the criteria for PTSD (APA, 1987). As noted earlier, this suggests that the levels of use of, or the need for, conventional psychiatric and related services should not be relied upon solely to understand the service requirements of, and the impact on, populations affected by violence. Tomlinson (2007) wondered, if services had adapted to the needs of those traumatised by the Troubles (i.e. if services had been developed to respond to the trauma and related needs), then would this have yielded different results? The experiences of the work in Omagh, the subject of this book, revealed that most often referrals for psychiatric care (i.e. secondary-level services) are channelled through self referral and frontline services (mainly family doctors). It is more than likely that a lot of initial distress and enduring psychological difficulties following traumatic events were managed by individuals, families and frontline services and therefore would not be picked up in studies looking at patterns of service use in secondary care. Finally, the review points to the need to ensure that the right questions are asked of those who suffer from experiences of violence and conflict. At least one study demonstrated that assessments based on PTSD criteria revealed greater need than conventional psychiatric assessments (Kee et al., 1987; Bell et al., 1988).

Gallagher (1987) came to related conclusions. First, he remarked that researchers were not asking all the appropriate questions about the violence and its impact. He observed that early researchers had focused on individual psychological effects and, finding few such effects, concluded that there were few social effects. He argued for research informed by Social Identity Theory (Tajfel, 1981). Cairns and colleagues took up this challenge and began to produce results demonstrating that the personal perceptions of violence were somehow related to people's psychological state, and that distancing (denial) played a part in helping many people to live within a community in violent conflict (e.g. Cairns and Wilson, 1991; Wilson and Cairns, 1992; Campbell et al. 2004).

The use of the GHQ in many of the studies discussed above provided a means of objectively and systematically understanding the well-being of the population in the face of violence. It allowed comparisons between, for example, those who had experienced, or had lived in areas, affected by violence and those who had not. It also enabled comparisons with other countries (chiefly England, Wales, Scotland and the Republic of Ireland), although here there is need for some caution. In the absence of baseline data (i.e. the position before the Troubles erupted), the position of Northern Ireland at any point thereafter lacks an anchor point of reference.

This problem showed up in the international comparisons first published by the NICTT-UU partnership (Ferry et al., 2008). Before the Troubles, the level of exposure to traumatic experiences within the Northern Irish population seemed to be below the mean for western advanced economies (Galea et al., 2005). One explanation is that, prior to the Troubles breaking out in the late 1960s, Northern Ireland was, relatively speaking, a low-trauma society characterised by religious and cultural conservatism and was much more agrarian than industrialised compared with many other developed countries. Also, the Troubles may, to one degree or another, have displaced the traumas found more commonly in settled industrialised and advanced societies. The risky behaviours of young men in non-conflict contexts were replaced by engagement in one or other form of aggressive or defensive activities in the Troubles.

On the question of methods, Loughrey and Curran (1987) envisaged the developing concept and diagnostic category of PTSD as having promise for researchers and practitioners. They saw the need for and benefit of a way of consistently classifying people's psychological difficulties that were consequential to traumatic experiences. This would create a level playing field and allow need to be understood objectively and systematically. The diverse experiences of people affected by their traumatic experiences could be understood and calibrated within a commonly agreed framework. If this were possible, then research could be carried out looking specifically at the needs of communities affected by common stressors such as the Troubles, and as demonstrated by the NICTT-UU series of studies, to compare findings across national boundaries.

The concept is also very relevant in a therapeutic context. The experiences of the Omagh Community Trauma and Recovery Team and the NICTT have demonstrated that people seeking help with a complicated, ill-defined and often devastating set of problems can feel enormous relief if their problems can be understood within a concept such as PTSD. Further, having such a tool equips the person seeking help to engage, with a clearer sense of the goals of therapy, with a perspective on what else needs to change to bring about improvements, and with a sense of hope for future recovery. Key to its value in research and in therapy is to see it as a tool, or a metaphor or a window through which people's experiences and needs can be helpfully understood. It goes without saying, but should nonetheless be said, that the value of such tools is that they are used empathetically and flexibly, mindful of the importance of the therapeutic relationship; also, that people who do not meet the set criteria might also be in great distress and have service and other needs.

Several studies point to the late onset of problems some time after the initial loss or trauma, referred to as latency. This seems to be more the case with anxiety disorders, of which PTSD is a kind. As mentioned above, the fact that people with anxiety disorders take an average of twenty-two years to seek help, has almost certainly contributed to the findings of greater need in later studies.

The work of the Consultative Group on the Past (Eames et al., 2009) identified the mental health consequences related to the losses and trauma of the Troubles as a distinctive component of a complex range of issues that require attention in post-conflict Northern Ireland. By doing so, they raised mental health issues, and the adverse effects of the civil conflict on mental health, to the level of social justice in a post-conflict context. This gives rise to the argument that mental health should be assessed as a key priority in the context of peace talks and political settlements, an issue that is discussed further in the following chapters.

From research to policy to services

As illustrated, the evidence from research and consultations into the impact of the Troubles was used to develop policy advice both in relation to health and social care measures, and in relation to areas specific to the needs of victims and survivors and their communities (e.g. DHSSPS, 2003; DHSSPS, 2007; Eames et al., 2009; OFMDFM, 2009). Whilst much has been done and resources deployed, at the time of writing, further development of policy and services, designed to respond to the evidence from research, is needed. Research in itself is essential, but not in itself sufficient, to bring about change and development in policy and in services. In societies not affected by conflict, the development of new or enhanced services requires service commissioning and funding decisions and, often, political actions that respond courageously and intelligently to evidence. In a post-conflict society where death, injury and trauma take the debate way beyond the facts and figures, the task for service commissioners, funders and politicians is even more challenging, but all the more necessary if people are to get access to the services they need. Further, as has been illustrated, such action is necessary to ensure that destructive narratives in the trauma and loss of individuals, families and communities who have been adversely affected by violence, and that are at the foundation of the passing conflict, are not carried forward into new generations.

Conclusions

This and the previous chapter have charted a pathway from the early days of the Troubles and the efforts to understand the mental health impact of the violence. The overview has used selected studies and the work of particular initiatives and groups to illustrate that effort, and to highlight key findings and learning points along the way. Other important and valuable studies, not reviewed here due to restrictions on space, would add much to this assessment, and benefit will be derived from further research which reveals more about needs and the mechanism that underlie those needs. For now, perhaps the key message is that, in spite of early hopes that the violence did not have a major impact, over time it has been discovered that many people have been adversely affected by direct and indirect experiences of violence, and that the consequences have since been felt and observed in later generations.

6

The Northern Ireland Centre for Trauma and Transformation: a comprehensive trauma centre

This chapter describes the origins of the Northern Ireland Centre for Trauma and Transformation (NICTT). It briefly outlines the philosophical and theoretical foundations of the Centre and the evidence base upon which its mission and work was developed. Each of the key areas of work is briefly outlined. The role of a not-for-profit agency working in conventional public sector funding and administrative structures in the context of the Troubles is briefly described.

Background to the NICTT

As described in Chapter 2, the original Omagh Community Trauma and Recovery Team was established immediately following the bombing in August 1998 and operated until 2001. During this period, over 600 people approached or were referred to the Team for help, mainly with psychological problems linked to their experiences of the bombing. Considerable experience was gained in responding to a community tragedy, on how to respond to the needs of people affected by traumatic events, and how to establish a trauma-focused psychosocial service for people with adverse psychological problems.

The therapy staff in particular developed experience and skills in relating to the trauma-needs of people who were seeking help. Having a sound basis for developing services, and access to research-based advice and support, was central to the establishment of the Team's trauma-focused service. Specifically, this included the pre-bomb work and experiences of the Team's clinical lead in the development and delivery of cognitive behavioural therapy (CBT), and the prior experiences of the Team manager in delivering and managing mental health and disability services. As discussed above, the research-based advice and support of Professor David Clark and colleagues at Oxford University was key to the early development of a trauma-focused approach and provided essential clinical support, especially in the early months after the bombing.

One of the key aims of the Sperrin Lakeland Trust, which established the Team, was to evaluate its experience and work, and to share as widely as possible the knowledge gained. In keeping with this aim, the Team's therapeutic work with people who suffered as a consequence of the bombing was reviewed. This took the form of an audit of patients with PTSD who were treated using the Ehlers-Clark (2000) trauma-focused approach to PTSD and related disorders. This audit is described in Chapter 5 (Gillespie et al., 2002).

The number of people seeking help from the Team declined in 2000. At this point, between two and three years after the bombing, the number of people with very acute problems and trauma-related symptoms had, as expected, reduced. Occasionally some would make contact with an acute traumatic reaction, either because something in the community associated with the bombing or something in their personal lives seemed to have provoked it. However, most of those seeking help by this point had been struggling with problems for some time. These had become deep-seated, and those seeking help were most usually presenting with more than one psychological disorder or life problem. The Team had the evidence from the four community needs-assessments described in Chapter 3, which suggested that significant numbers of adults and children might yet seek help with psychological problems related to their experience of the bombing. It was expected that there would be a need for a sustained specialist trauma-focused service for some time to come, although involving lower numbers than in the first few months after the bombing.

The original strategy for the Community Trauma and Recovery Team to the bombing had envisaged an end to the special and additional measures that were put in place to respond to the bombing (Bolton, 1998). It was not clear at the outset when this point would be reached. It had originally been the view that when the numbers of referrals to the Team fell to a level that could be managed within the mainstream public mental health services and not-for-profit sector in the Omagh community, then that was the point at which the Team should close. The strategy had been reviewed annually, and at the third review the decision was made to consult with the wider community and other individuals and agencies beyond Omagh that had an interest in or concern for the continuing needs of those affected by the bombing, on the future provision of specialist trauma services.

The expectancy of an end to the work, built into the plans for the Community Trauma and Recovery Team's workload from the outset, and indeed the plans for the wider response by the Sperrin Lakeland Trust, was a helpful and important feature of the planning for the response to the bombing. Philosophically, it conveyed and reinforced the expectancy that a time would come when, in spite of the terrible losses and experiences suffered by individuals and families, and by the community as a whole, a level of resilience and mastery over the tragedy would be reached. It also made clear from the beginning that the service would come to an end, thereby shaping expectations about services and funding in the longer-term. This was an important point for funders who knew they were funding a finite commitment.

Consulting on the future provision of services

All the same, the enduring needs of some individuals, and the as yet unknown and unexpressed needs of others, provided the basis for conversations as to when the Team should close and what, if anything, should be put in its place. A further consideration was whether anything should be done to build upon the unique experiences and skills of the Trauma and Recovery Team in responding to the bombing. To explore opinion on these matters, the chief executive of the Sperrin Lakeland Trust wrote to organisations and individuals involved in the response to the bombing, or otherwise concerned with the Omagh community, to consult on the future provision of specialist trauma services, and what, if anything, should happen next.

Those who were consulted were from a wide range of community interests who had, in one way or another, been involved in the work and life of the Team and who were concerned for various reasons with the impact of the bombing on the community. They included individuals and families who had been affected by the bombing; government departments; public bodies with responsibility for the commissioning of services; and those concerned with providing the services. The key objective was to ensure that people who had been affected by the Omagh bombing, and who had yet to come forward for help, would have access to trauma-focused services of the kind that had been provided by the Team. The support of those consulted in relation to the timing of the closure was important to ensure those in the community who still had problems would not feel they had no recourse to help should they need it.

The consultation showed there was general acceptance that, with the reduction in referrals to the Team, it should close, on the condition that there would continue to be access to specialist trauma services. In relation to what should be done to harness and build upon the experiences and skills developed by the Team, almost all of those consulted supported the development of a further initiative that would extend trauma services of the kind developed in Omagh to the wider population. The consultation had also confirmed that whilst capability had been built up within local services in the wake of the bombing, there would remain a need for specialist provision to address the needs of those who had yet to seek help and who had more complex needs. This, in particular, was a matter of concern for the Omagh Fund, the chairman and trustees of which were anxious to ensure that services were sustained as long as possible for those affected by the bombing and who might not at that point have sought help.

Responders wished to see steps that would harness the experience developed in the wake of the bombing for the wider benefit of those who had suffered from the years of violence in both Northern Ireland and in the border region of the Republic of Ireland. In particular, they thought that the experience acquired, and the knowledge and skills developed, in understanding, assessing and addressing the psychological impact of the tragedy should be retained for the wider benefit of the population. Quite a few responders, inspired by the generosity shown by many across Ireland and the wider world in response to the Omagh bombing, thought efforts should be made to share the experience of developing trauma services with other communities affected by tragedies. Finally, staff who had worked in the Community Trauma and Recovery Team wanted what had been learned, developed and achieved taken forward, and some were interested in being part of a new initiative, beyond the work of the Team.

Evidence of the need for a new service

The original Omagh Community Trauma and Recovery Team had involved practitioners from a wide range of roles and disciplines (from mental health, disability services, administration and managerial backgrounds) and was directly linked into the wider range of services provided by the Sperrin Lakeland Trust (including hospital and community services). The Team was also connected with the work of local family doctors, mental health services and not-for-profit and community organisations. It had connections and interactions, particularly in the first two years, with education services and schools and a wide range of interests and groups in the community. Taking a psycho-social approach, its focus was on therapeutic services for individuals and families, and on wider community recovery. It also paid attention to issues relevant to the management of a tragedy that had arisen from a politically motivated act of violence. This involved routine connections with politicians and policy-makers, as well as offering comment on political issues that had a bearing on the health and related needs of service users. In the context of a single community tragedy associated with the Troubles and with this configuration and connections, the Team was part of a unique and comprehensive community located system.

As described in Chapter 3, after the bombing, four major needs-assessments were undertaken into its impact in order to inform future service needs. The highly valuable information derived from the studies pointed to the level of need in the community following the bombing. The studies described the impact of a single atrocity in the context of the many atrocities of the years of violence. So it was possible, in general terms, to infer from the Omagh bombing example, what the wider need arising from the Troubles might be. It was concluded that the data and conclusions of the studies were strong evidence of the extensive impact of violence linked to the conflict. This conclusion pointed to the benefit of using the experience of addressing the needs of those affected by the Omagh bombing, in the service of the wider community.

Addressing mental health needs as part of peace-making

The development of ideas about recognising the mental health impact of the Troubles, and responding effectively, was part of a wider debate about addressing the adverse impact of the years of violence on individuals, families and communities (e.g. Bloomfield, 1998). More widely, this theme formed part of the consideration of wider discussions and theorising as to what it takes for a society that has been affected by civil conflict to make peace, build peace and be transformed into a new stable entity. Much of this discussion was associated with the European Union's Peace programmes, established by the European Commission in 1995 following the first cease-fires (Hughes, 2011).

The clear conclusion of the consultations about the future development of services based upon the early work in Omagh was that something should be developed beyond the early work, as a humanitarian response to the psychological and mental health needs of people affected by violence. The developing ideas were also supported, to some extent, on the basis that responding to the trauma- and grief-related needs of communities affected by violence was an essential part of the victims-focused reparation tasks, which in turn formed part of the wider task of peace-making and peace-building (e.g. McGarry and O'Leary, 1993; Lederach, 1998).

Practical steps towards new proposals

The experience and research from the original Team's work highlighted the specialist service requirements of people suffering severe and chronic trauma-related disorders. As a result, and in view of the comments of those who responded to the consultation on future services, it was clear that the focus of the new initiative should be on the further development and delivery of trauma-focused therapy services for the wider population of people suffering trauma-related disorders. This focus addressed the very apparent gap in the range of services available for those who were suffering longer-term with the complicated psychological and mental health consequences of their experiences.

Building on the consultations across the community, conversations took place between Omagh District Council, the Sperrin Lakeland Trust and the Trust's main service commissioner, the Western Health and Social Services Board. This led to the commissioning of a feasibility study on the preliminary ideas and proposals for the next steps. There were also discussions with the Victims Liaison Unit, the unit within the Northern Ireland Office with responsibility for the development of services for individuals and communities affected by the Troubles. At the time, the unit was developing policy and services in response to the recommendations of the Victims Commissioner (Bloomfield, 1998).

Decisions about the areas to be addressed under the new proposals

At this early stage, and particularly on the basis of the feedback from the local community, the view was building, that any new initiative should be established as an autonomous body, separate from the public health services. There were several drivers for this view. One was that whatever emerged should be in some way linked to Omagh and almost certainly based there. It was thought that incorporating the new development within the public sector would leave it liable to being changed by wider forces and pressures. This sentiment was linked to a debate underway at the time on the future of the local hospital, which had given rise to much disquiet in the Omagh community. Second, there were concerns that when the memory of the significance of the work undertaken in Omagh was fading, the initiative would be vulnerable to financial and other organisational pressures. Third, the support from the public sector for the new development was mixed and it was thought that the development might suffer from a lack of support at the important early stages or again could be vulnerable to changing priorities. It was also thought that the configuration of the proposed service (envisaged to incorporate research, training and humanitarian relief, as well as service provision) would not fit well within a public service whose focus was chiefly service delivery. Finally, it was thought that in being autonomous and independent, the new development could draw in funding from non-public, philanthropic and other grants-based sources, as well as public funding. So having an independent status would probably strengthen prospects of the long-term sustainability.

To assist subsequent discussions, and to reflect the emerging views and ideas, a set of proposals were developed which envisaged a range of services being provided by a new independent organisation. This developed into the vision of a Centre, established by an autonomous body separate from, but with vital links with, public services, anchored in the Omagh community, yet reaching out to the wider population and beyond. Based upon the experience of the original Omagh Team, and on the comments received in response to the consultation, it was determined that the new service should have at its core four primary programmes, namely the delivery of trauma-focused psychological therapies; research; training; and humanitarian relief. (Later, based on the early experiences of the new Centre, a fifth programme, advocacy and policy support, was added.)

Research-based theory for trauma centres

Around this time, the process had the benefit of a new publication. Williams and Nurmi (2001) had investigated and reported upon 66 trauma centres across the world and summarised from their findings the key features, cultures, characteristics and services of what they referred to as 'a comprehensive trauma center'.

Williams and Nurmi's work became available as the development work on the establishment of the Centre was concluding, offering a key reference, plus a set of principles and characteristics, against which the proposals could be tested. It was clear that the proposals met Williams and Nurmi's criteria for the core activities within a comprehensive trauma centre (i.e. therapy services, research and training) with additional features relevant to the history and context in which the proposals had been developed (advocacy and policy, and humanitarian relief). The publication reinforced the conclusions that had emerged from the Omagh community consultations and from the experience of the original Trauma and Recovery Team, providing further valuable insights, principles, and areas for attention and caution.

The proposals

Key to taking these ideas forward was the securing of funding. On the basis of this work and analysis, in 2001 a proposal was made to the Northern Ireland Office for the funding of the new Centre. As noted earlier, the policy context at the time was that the Northern Ireland Office was endeavouring to implement the Victims Commissioner's recommendations (Bloomfield, 1998). Evidence from the audit (Gillespie et al., 2002) of therapy for patients suffering PTSD undertaken by the Trauma and Recovery Team provided crucial evidence to support the proposals, along with evidence of the demand for services and the implications of chronic disorders arising from traumatic experiences. The new Centre would focus on psychological trauma. The rationale was that it would build upon the three-and-a-half years' experience of the original Community Trauma and Recovery Team. It would extend the provision of trauma-focused therapies provided by the original Omagh Team to people in the wider Northern Ireland population who had been adversely affected by the Troubles. Its specialist therapy would also be available to those affected by the Omagh bombing who had yet to seek help. The Centre would undertake research, and develop training and education programmes to support the development of trauma-focused skills and practices within the public and not-for-profit sectors. Through its humanitarian programme the Centre would reach out to other communities affected by conflict and share the work and experience developed at Omagh with those interested in developing their own trauma-focused services. Finally, the Centre would work in partnership with other agencies at local, regional and international levels.

Governance arrangements

Once it became clear that the proposals were likely to be supported, work began to establish a charitable (not-for-profit) trust, which would form the governing body for the new Centre. Five members of the public active in public life in Northern Ireland and the Republic of Ireland, some with strong links to Omagh and the Omagh tragedy, and with business, mental health, therapy and other relevant backgrounds and skills, were invited to form the governing body. This shadow trust sought charitable status and put in place the managerial and governance arrangements to support the establishment of the Centre and the management of funds. The trustees decided that the new Centre should be known as The Northern Ireland Centre for Trauma and Transformation (NICTT) and commissioned its logo from the artist who had led the Petals of Hope initiative in Omagh following the bombing (described in Chapter 1). They also decided that the Centre's mission should be, 'Treating Trauma – Advancing knowledge – Contributing to Transformation'. One of the ambitions the trustees had for the new Centre was that it would contribute to the positive transformation of the lives of individuals and of the wider community. They wished to convey the hope that trauma in the lives of individuals and communities was not inevitable and could be overcome. Hence, the word 'transformation' featured in the title and in the mission statement of the new organization, and became an important reference point for the trustees.

Connecting the new service with existing services

Further conversations with key agencies took place to ensure that they were acquainted with the details of the proposals and to obtain any views they had on how best the Centre could operate and fit into the wider service landscape. Overwhelmingly, the proposals were met with enthusiasm, and with a general agreement that there was a need for a specialist trauma centre that could work in support of mainstream services and act as a driver for developing practice and services. The basis for the new Centre had been established in the three-and-a-half years' experience of the original Omagh Community Trauma and Recovery Team, which had provided new insights into the scale and nature of the impact that the conflict-related violence had on the mental health of the population. Also, the original work of the Team had been the subject of a formal audit (subsequently published in a peer reviewed paper) as to the effectiveness of the new trauma-focused methods developed after the Omagh bombing. The new Centre's establishment represented a significant financial investment in service development, upon which future services could be built.

Accommodation

It was decided that the Centre would be located in rented property and work began on finding suitable premises. The reasons for this were that buying property would have been a challenge in itself (i.e. raising the capital and managing the purchasing, modification or building of premises). Whilst premises could become an asset, a building would have also brought with it liabilities and would reduce manoeuvrability in the event that the Centre or the trustees wished to make significant changes, to take account of either reduced or increased future funding. At this early stage it was unclear what the best configuration for the delivery of services should be, so again, ownership of a building would have reduced flexibility.

The new Centre opens

In May 2002 the new Centre opened in Omagh. Around the same time, the Northern Ireland Government published its strategy for addressing the needs of victims of the violence (OFMDFM, 2002), which located the new Centre's ambitions and contribution in a wider policy framework. Key staff who had worked in the original Omagh Team were recruited to the new Centre, including the Team's clinical lead and team manager. Over the following months additional therapists and support staff were added to the Centre's staff. To achieve this progress involved significant efforts by the trustees of the NICTT Trust, with support from the Sperrin Lakeland Trust and with decisions being acted upon by the Centre's business and development manager.

The therapy programme

Work commenced to develop the trauma-focused CBT service for people affected by the years of violence in Northern Ireland (Ehlers and Clark; 2000; discussed further in Chapter 7). Over the following ten years the service received over 700 referrals, a number limited only by commitments to the Centre's training and research programme. The work of the Centre revealed a significant need for specialist trauma services and showed that once offered, people suffering trauma-related disorders would refer themselves, or be referred for help.

The research programme

Work also commenced on developing the Centre's research programme. Two key areas of research were identified as being important for the development of services. First, the aim was to better understand how effective the Centre's therapeutic approach was in addressing chronic trauma disorders arising from conflict. This led to a randomised controlled trial, which is described in more detail in Chapter 9. The second was to investigate the population impact of the years of violence. There were several localised or group focused studies, including the four community needs-assessments undertaken in the Omagh area after the 1998 bombing (Chapter 3). However, it was difficult to infer with confidence from these as to what the wider population impact was of the violence and its longer-term consequences. The lack of a comprehensive population-wide epidemiological study of the impact of the Troubles had already been noted as necessary by a number of observers (Daly, 1999; Deloitte and Touche, 2003). This, coupled with the Centre's experiences of the Omagh tragedy and in delivering trauma-focused services to Troubles-affected communities and groups, reinforced the Centre's aims of undertaking such a study.

The training and education programme

The Centre's aims included the development of training and education programmes focusing on trauma-related courses to advance knowledge and skills about trauma. In time this work included briefings on the findings of the clinical team on its experiences and the therapeutic challenges and outcomes in serving a wider and much more chronic population suffering trauma-related disorders. To support policy change and advocate for service improvements, these briefings were provided for politicians; government departments; governmental and non-governmental agencies and officials; various intermediary and umbrella organisations working to address the impact of the years of violence; funders; and a wide range of groups and interests working in the community. During the life of the Centre several hundred such briefings were provided. These afforded opportunities for others to hear about and learn from the experience of the Centre and its predecessor, the Omagh Community Trauma and Recovery Team. The key content included data about the range and severity of the needs of those who had experienced violence and consequently suffered adverse psychological and mental health consequences. The briefings provided evidence of the need for specialist trauma therapy provision and the necessity of having the wider health and social care systems being activated to identify, support and refer people with severe trauma-related needs. They also provided valuable opportunities to hear from the range of government, public and not-for-profit agencies and individuals on their experiences and views. These exchanges influenced the Centre's therapy services, the type of training that it was developing, and the focus of its research.

Beyond these briefings, the Centre began to explore the interest in and need for training in methods aimed at effectively treating trauma-related disorders. Over the ten years of the Centre's operations, an integrated programme of training was developed and delivered. Initially, the training was informal and unaccredited. This enabled some experimentation with teaching methods, and an exploration of the areas of interest and training deficits of service providers and practitioners. Later, academic training was developed at Ulster University in collaboration with the Team manager of the Centre who had left to take up a post there as a senior lecturer. This involved a joint Postgraduate Certificate and Masters qualification in Cognitive Therapy, the Masters including a specialist module on treating PTSD. Later, and with confidence drawn from earlier experiences, and especially from teaching in Sri Lanka and Bosnia, a series of short vocational courses were developed to raise awareness and enhance skills in relation to trauma needs and therapeutic practice. This work is described in more detail in Chapter 8.

Funding and funding challenges

For the first three-and-a-half years, the Centre was funded to deliver its core activities (therapy, research and training) by the Northern Ireland Office, which was responsible for the governance of Northern Ireland pending the establishment of a new local administration. It had been intended that this initial investment in the Centre would be a pump primer for the development of services, the building of knowledge through research, and skills through training and education. These activities would support the wider development of services for those who had suffered adversely from mental health problems linked to the Troubles.

Funding was provided by the Omagh Fund, through which additional trauma-focused services were made available to people adversely affected by the Omagh bombing. The Centre's humanitarian work and research were funded through specific grants from other donors linked to those activities. Over its lifetime, the trustees and the Centre secured additional funding for these and other projects, adding value to the governmental funding – one of the advantages of a partnership between government and the independent sector. More often than not, independent funders were interested in funding additional programmes that complemented the core activities of the Centre e.g. additional therapeutic services, research and capacity building. Independent funders were attracted by the commitment of government agencies.

During the first three-and-a-half years of the Centre's life, local governmental structures and institutions were re-established in Belfast with the formation of a new Assembly and Executive – all part of the unfolding political progress. Thereafter, until it closed in 2011, the Centre secured further funding through various structures in the new local administration. This was essential for the continued delivery of services, in particular the trauma therapy programme. During this period, funding became increasingly short-term, which posed particular problems for the recruitment and retention of highly skilled therapists. More positively, the Centre's initial costs, for what was in the early days a research and development institute, were being reduced as this phase of the Centre's work paved the way for more routine delivery of therapy services. Established relationships, and the development of a reputation with independent funders, enabled additional activities such as research and training to be undertaken.

Closure and further dissemination of the learning

Short funding horizons, the loss of key staff, and the ending of funding for core activities led to the decision by the trustees to close the Centre at the end of 2011. The principal consideration was the service and safety issues in providing therapy for a group of patients, many of whom had long-term and complicated needs. Regrettable though the decision was, the trustees considered it best to close the Centre in a managed way and where possible to find alternatives for patients who had been referred to the Centre.

The process of closure itself was a complex undertaking, with considerable logistical and governance implications. For instance, arrangements had to be made for the destruction or retention of records, for the disposal of property and the ending of leases, and for ensuring obligations to staff were met. Partners and agencies involved in the life of the Centre had to be informed. This work continued for a period following the closure of the doors of the Centre. Importantly, the trustees had, in earlier years, set aside funds for administering the closure and proper winding up of the Centre.

Mindful of the heritage of the Centre's work and achievements over ten years the Centre's trustees made decisions to ensure that wherever and however possible the lessons it had learned should be made widely available. The trustees continued to operate as a governing body to take this forward. One such initiative included a knowledge transfer programme with Northern Ireland's Victims and Survivors Service with the support of the Research and Development Division of Northern Ireland's Public Health Agency. Having overseen the closure of the Centre and putting in place arrangements for the dissemination of its work and learning, the trustees wound up the Centre's governing trust in 2015.

Conclusions

Setting up and maintaining an organisation to address the mental health impacts of conflict posed considerable challenges. One of these is legitimacy, especially in a context where there are different, often polarised or competing views on what should be done to address such needs. The lack of previous initiatives in response to particular incidents, or the Troubles in general, meant that there was some reluctance to develop services. It was deemed people with needs already had access to conventional services. In Northern Ireland, the civil conflict was as much a psychological conflict, part of the armoury of terrorism. The killing of one person could have major communal repercussions, and such acts were often intended to achieve this effect. At times it felt as though setting up services to redress the psychological impacts of acts of terror and other conflict-related violence was being interpreted as a measure aimed at rolling back the intentional terrorisation they caused. The anxiety this caused must have played its part over the years of the Troubles in inhibiting service developments. There can be lots of reasons for doing nothing. Stepping beyond such considerations, and the fears they give rise to, is only the start.

The work developed in Omagh immediately after the bombing was both spontaneous and inevitable because of the scale of the bombing, its timing just after the Belfast Agreement, and the potential implications of the bombing for the peace process. The later development of the NICTT was linked directly to the lessons learned in the white heat of the Omagh bombing tragedy. The early work had generated a body of evidence, which supported the need for new and increased levels of services for those who had been affected by the Troubles. Other research around the same time was reaching similar conclusions (see Chapter 5). Those consulted on the future of the original Omagh Community Trauma and Recovery Team, widely supported a new initiative that would make what was learnt after the bombing more widely available. The proposed configuration of the new Centre was designed to reflect the lessons learned, the evidence, and the aspirations of the Omagh community. The proposals were directly relevant to government policy, which was essential for primary funding. Theoretically, the configuration of the NICTT was supported by the concept of the Comprehensive Trauma Centre developed by Williams and Nurmi (2001). The trustees of the new NICTT brought with them deep connections into the life of the community, with skills and experiences highly relevant to the proposed work of the Centre. Staff who had worked in the original Team and moved to the new Centre brought with them a unique set of skills and capabilities, backed up by national and international academic and other resources. The not-for-profit arrangements for the new Centre allowed it to be flexible and innovative, and to make connections and interfaces between different areas of knowledge and experience. This had the ultimate aim of delivering a body of research, competences and skills that could be mainstreamed eventually into public services. Yet, even with these strengths and possibilities, the Centre faced considerable challenges in making its way.

Amongst its accomplishments over ten years of operation, the Centre's therapy and research programmes revealed that there was a significant need and demand for access by the public to specialist trauma-focused therapeutic services. It also revealed that practitioners and agencies wanted training in trauma awareness and skills, and the Centre put in place appropriate programmes to respond to these aspirations. Its research into needs and services contributed to the knowledge base, which was made widely available to inform and support policy. This included offering evidence and analyses that – in the context of conflict – politicians, political parties and others, such as therapeutic service providers and practitioners, could build upon. The Centre's work also provided data and practice-based information and experiences that could inform and shape service commissioning, service delivery and practice. Perhaps of greatest significance, it delivered services to many hundreds of people who had been adversely affected by the Troubles, bringing help, support and recovery.

The Centre faced the common challenge of small mission-driven organisations to secure funding from a range of funders to support its endeavours, given that a single funder was unlikely to fund all of its programmes. As already noted, philanthropic and grant-making funders tended to be interested in supporting time-limited projects that added value to the core work of the Centre. Core services that would ideally have been available routinely to the public were considered by independent funders to be the responsibility of government and related funders. As an innovator the Centre from time to time acquired project funding, for instance to support its efforts to share what it had learned. An example was early project funding for training through the European Union Interreg IIIA and Peace II programmes, which supported capacity building within the wider workforce (Fee, 2008).

The experience of the Centre illustrates again that not-for-profit organisations can deliver specialist services. This necessarily requires sensible levels of funding over sensible periods that will enable them to recruit, retain and support skilled staff to ensure that a specialist service is available on a consistent basis. In this instance, some of the difficulties related to difficulties in political progress, which resulted in stop-go funding, one of the challenges of operating a service in a fractious post-conflict political environment. Policy advisers and makers, service commissioners and funders have a key role to play in helping to overcome such problems by understanding and advocating for the role of specialist therapy and other services in the context of a needs-led and stepped-care system, especially where innovation is required to address poorly understood or emerging needs such as those linked to the Troubles.

7

The development of a trauma-focused therapy programme

This chapter describes the establishment of a trauma-focused approach to the needs of those seeking help with emotional, psychological and mental health problems linked to traumatic experiences of the civil conflict in Northern Ireland. The chapter will outline the development of a therapy service based upon trauma-focused cognitive behavioural therapy (CBT). Key issues relating to the origins, principles, aims and challenges of this development will be described and discussed.

As described in Chapter 6, by 2001 the number of people affected by the Omagh bombing who were being referred to the Omagh Community Trauma and Recovery Team had reduced considerably, so much so that the Team was reducing in size. After extensive consultations, and in line with the original strategy for responding to the bombing (Bolton, 1998), the decision was taken to close the Team in 2001. The consultations were followed by the establishment of a new organisation, the Northern Ireland Centre for Trauma and Transformation (NICTT), with the aim of building upon the earlier work for the benefit of the wider population affected by the Troubles. The new Centre's programmes were to deliver trauma therapies, undertake research, train practitioners in trauma-related skills, and support other communities affected by war and conflict. The Centre opened in May 2002 and closed in December 2011.

Laying the foundations

The therapeutic work of the new Centre focused on trauma-related disorders linked to the Troubles. In view of its origins, the therapy service was intended to be for adults only, although children could become involved with their parents' therapy sessions or other meetings within the Centre. It was clear that the Centre should work with patients using the trauma-focused CBT developed in the original Omagh Community Trauma and Recovery Team (Ehlers and Clark, 2000; Gillespie et al., 2002). Importantly, a small but growing group of experienced practitioners, some of whom were contributing to training and supervision in CBT, had also been developed within the public sector services.

The original Omagh Team had included a range of therapists from various health and social care backgrounds. Ideally, if there had been sufficient resources, this more broadly based team could have been reproduced in the new Centre. However, limited resources was an unavoidable consideration – although new developments in support services for victims and survivors meant that the Centre was able to connect with publicly funded mental health, rehabilitatory and support services. A more significant matter, however, was the absence of, and therefore the need for, specialist provision in trauma therapy that would offer a level of service not routinely available previously. The new Centre's specialist service would connect, where required, with other mental health, rehabilitatory and support services – some of which might, had funding been available, been otherwise incorporated into a more extensive and integrated organisation.

Trauma-focused CBT

Central to decisions about the work and focus of the new Centre was the knowledge that trauma-focused CBT offered an approach that was effective with trauma-related disorders. Importantly, through the work of the original Omagh Team it had been demonstrated that the approach was particularly relevant and effective for people who had suffered as a consequence of the Troubles. Pivotally, patients generally liked the approach, engaging with it effectively and enthusiastically, bringing to the therapy their own resources and insights. Patients showed considerable progress, with reductions in their symptoms, assumptions of post-trauma lives that had meaning and fulfilment, and the resumption of family, social and economic roles. Moreover, it was clear that the approach could be highly centred on and adaptable to the unique needs of each individual, to the challenging context of civil conflict, and to the intense and chronic community tragedy it created. This, in the context of a long-lasting conflict, was particularly relevant to the many who had suffered trauma-related disorders over many years. With finite resources and the limited availability of a trauma-focused therapeutic service, it was better to invest what was available in a focused approach underpinned by a strong and developing evidence base and with an already developed capability at local level. Further, it was important that there was the capability to extend the number of practitioners and further develop skills and supervision at a highly skilled level. This was necessary so that the capacity to deliver a trauma-focused range of services for a conflict-affected population with increasingly complex needs was increased from relatively low levels in the community to a level required to meet the unfolding needs of the population. Finally, it was also clear that the Centre should continue to evaluate and learn from the needs and views of patients and families and from the experiences of delivering a trauma service.

As described in Chapter 2, the trauma-focused CBT approach was based upon the work of Ehlers and Clark (2000). The approach was relevant because of its specificity to trauma-related disorders including PTSD. Ehlers and Clark's contribution brought a precision of concept and language to the consideration of traumatic experiences and their consequences. Their work provided a description of the interconnecting components of trauma and a cognitive behavioural approach to understanding and treating trauma disorders. Helpfully, they described and differentiated the key behavioural and cognitive components that maintained PTSD. They also described how these relate to the characteristics of traumatic memories and to the environmental and other external and internal triggers that precipitate distressing recollections of the traumatic event, such as flashbacks. In short, they described what it is about traumatic experiences that cause some people thereafter to have distressing and puzzling psychological feelings and thoughts. They also described what it is about how we respond to and manage the distressing memories of events that can maintain traumatic reactions – even though initially our responses and behaviours were efforts to manage the distress. From there they described what can be done therapeutically to address the unhelpful cognitive and behavioural responses to the distress of traumatic experiences – thereby enabling recovery. Through their research and development Ehlers, Clark and colleagues demonstrated that people suffering PTSD could benefit significantly from a trauma-focused cognitive behavioural therapeutic approach.

The 'trauma focus' is important to stress as this underlines the necessity of the therapist bringing that additional and essential set of considerations to the more generic CBT approach – or indeed any mode of therapy. For example, a person with PTSD receiving generic CBT might benefit somewhat from such an intervention. By bringing a trauma focus to the CBT, people suffering PTSD are likely to benefit much more.

CBT is a highly person-centred and collaborative approach to addressing psychological and related needs. It relies upon an active partnership between the patient and the therapist, and the idea of there being two experts in the room – one on the life experiences, capabilities, resources and needs of the patient, the other on the CBT approach. CBT draws its strengths from a set of principles, approaches and skills, yet in the hands of a competent practitioner is not a prescriptive approach and is highly adaptable to the unique needs of each individual.

Another innovation introduced by the team from Oxford to the work of the original Omagh Community Trauma and Recovery team, and later, the NICTT, was session-by-session outcome monitoring where patients completed standard mental health instruments (such as the BDI or PDS) at each therapy session. This was used in order to ensure that the needs and therapy outcomes of everyone who had treatment in NICTT would be known (Gillespie et al., 2002). At the time, this approach was not routine in mental health services, which meant there were often poor measures of need and therapeutic outcomes. The success in using session-by-session monitoring in Omagh later directly influenced key developments in other places, such as the Improving Access to Psychological Therapies Initiative in England (Clark, 2011), where (in 2016) IAPT achieved pre- and post-treatment measures of depression and anxiety from 98% of all patients who received a course of treatment through its programmes. (Correspondence with Professor David Clark, January 2017.)

This therapeutic approach, coupled with a trauma focus that had been demonstrated to be relevant to the needs of people affected by the conflict-related violence, opened up the possibility of developing a coherent and consistent service for people affected by the Troubles. Further, it could increasingly be scaled up in terms of skills and numbers of practitioners. It had also been demonstrated that the approach could handle the deep and very real anxieties of a population affected by violence and threats of violence. In spite of challenging external circumstances, such as on-going violence or threats to patients, the approach enabled the patient and the therapist to identify the therapeutic goals and priorities most relevant to those circumstances and the patient's current needs. Offering an irrelevant, untimely or ineffective service is clearly of no advantage to patients. It is also highly de-skilling and de-motivating for practitioners. Trauma-focused CBT was generally very well received by patients and, as evidenced from patient feedback, supervision, audit and research, made a significant positive impact on symptoms and enabled recovery.

This body of experience formed part of the evidence that led to the publication of advice on how to treat PTSD, first in 2003, with the publication of Northern Ireland's health department's guidance – on the management of PTSD in adults (DHSSPS, 2003). Later, in 2005, similar guidance on the management of PTSD in adults and children was issued by the National Institute for Health and Care Excellence (NICE, 2005).

Establishing the therapy team

The psychiatrist/CBT practitioner who had been the clinical lead in the original Omagh Team, along with the Team leader, moved to the new Centre, bringing with them much experience and highly developed skills in addressing trauma-related disorders. Importantly, they also brought a keen sense of the specific challenges of doing so in the context of conflict. Respectively, they took up the positions of clinical director and therapy team leader, and were later joined by one of the cognitive behavioural therapists involved in the original Omagh Team, plus other newly recruited cognitive behavioural therapists. Later, a social worker with extensive experience in family and child care, disability services and related areas joined the Centre to provide the first point of therapeutic contact for the public and to support the therapeutic work with individual patients in liaison with the therapists. A business development manager, administration staff and the director made up the rest of the Centre's team.

At an early stage, links were established by the Centre with family doctors and mental health services across Northern Ireland, as well as other agencies such as education services, faith communities, and providers in the not-for-profit and community sectors, chiefly to let them know about the new service and how to access it. In the context of the Troubles, links with organisations representing or working to support particular groups of people affected by violence was of particular importance. Referrals began to be received almost immediately, especially from services already familiar with the earlier work of the original Trauma and Recovery Team. Before long, people from outside the experience of the Omagh bombing began to access the Centre's new therapy service. It became clear from this wider patient group that there was, in the wider population, notable levels of enduring and chronic trauma-related disorders linked to experiences of the Troubles. It was learned early on that one of the most effective means by which patients learnt about the therapy service was from people they knew who had attended the Centre. During the years the therapy service was provided, a significant proportion of patients were referred, or referred themselves as a consequence of such personal contacts.

Member, patient, client or service user?

The term 'patient' was adopted as the preferred term to refer to those who sought help from the Centre. This was based principally upon consultations with people attending the original Omagh Community Trauma and Recovery Team for therapy, from which it was clear there was a robust majority for the term 'patient'. Compared to 'member' – a widely used term in the victims and survivors sector – the term 'patient' inferred a different relationship and at least hinted at a beginning and an end to the person's engagement with the Centre. The term was also thought by the Centre staff to be in accord with its use of its therapeutic approach, which, whilst not a medical intervention, was, all the same, a serious attempt to apply a scientific and evidence based approach to psychological and mental health disorders. For related reasons the terms 'client' and 'service users' were not used formally. There were also reasons for taking this approach linked to the role of the Centre in the context of conflict. The team took the view that the term 'patient' imparted a clear purpose to the work of the Centre in a context where patients or the Centre itself could be subject to threats or acts of violence. The term would be more likely to communicate the work and role of the Centre to those who might wish to obstruct its work, or threaten or attack the Centre itself or those attending it for therapy.

Accessing the therapy service

The Centre adopted an open door policy whereby anyone could refer themselves directly, as well as being referred by a relative or another individual or agency. This was unusual for a specialist therapy service but the Centre's team recognised how essential it is to have no obstacles in the way of people accessing help. This approach was introduced as a matter of principle in the original Omagh Team and was shown be essential to those struggling with trauma-related problems. Generally, it was found that individuals, or those close to them, were very capable of recognising their needs and it was therefore appropriate that they should have direct access to services – assuming that is, they knew about the Centre and its therapy programme. It was learned over time that the needs of those who referred themselves most often corresponded closely to the Centre's therapy programme. If they did not, people were sympathetically helped to access other more relevant services.

Typically, when people accessed the Centre, they presented with a mixture of heightened or distressing feelings and thoughts, physical responses and behaviours. They often came with concerns about the impact of how they felt on their relationships, family, social and economic lives. Through the initial assessment the therapist, in collaboration with the patient, tried to make sense of this amorphous mixture of experiences, problems and concerns. These clinical assessments involved the use of standardised instruments measuring trauma experiences, reactions, mood and anxiety including the PDS (Foa et al., 1997) and the BDI (Beck et al., 1988).

When therapists shared their view of the initial assessment with patients, typically patients responded with a great sense of relief. Sometimes, perhaps for the first time, the link between how people were feeling, thinking and behaving was associated with specific adverse events in their lives. This, and the fact that their needs were understood, that they had had similar experiences to others who had had traumatic experiences, and that they could be assisted through therapy, usually led to a marked improvement in their distress. The loneliness of the trauma sufferer, particularly before they are able to even think about seeking help, cannot be underestimated. Whereas people had previously felt very alone and beyond help, they now felt that their needs were not unique and that they could be helped. This had an immediate morale raising effect, which usually brought the patient immediately to a better place. Even if they continued to have considerable anxieties about discussing the unthinkable, patients were typically motivated to engage in therapy. It was found that if someone presented for assessment then the chances of continuing with therapy were very high. Key to this was the establishment of a relationship with the Centre and one of its therapy staff, and of having successfully taken that first step in crossing a threshold of anxiety and fear about addressing what was at its core a deeply troubling issue in their lives.

It was also necessary to help key care practitioners, such as family doctors, family members and employers, to know what to expect – and to be ready to support people through difficult times as therapy progressed.

The reluctance to talk about the unthinkable almost certainly has implications for whether and how victims of conflict-related violence pursue questions of justice relating to their experiences. It also suggests that many affected by violence are invisible to political and administration systems, and to services, directly because they will not and cannot present themselves as people with loss or trauma-related needs.

The biggest drop-out was at the pre-assessment stage, when people who were referred to the Centre (i.e. did not refer themselves) did not attend for assessment. Based on how difficult it is for people suffering trauma-related disorders, and in particular PTSD which includes avoidance, distancing and numbing amongst its qualifying symptoms (APA, 1994), the Centre's open referral policy was an essential feature. This was especially so as it was aimed at enabling as quick a response as possible where it seemed that people had sought help at a moment of crisis – after their previously successful, if unsustainable, methods of coping with the distress of their trauma, began to fail or collapsed.

Whilst the Centre was not an emergency service, from time to time people would refer themselves or be referred at a time of deep distress or anxiety. This included a number of enquirers who came to the Centre with little or no advance notice, desiring to see someone urgently, and usually in a state of deep distress. If a member of the therapy team was available then such callers were seen. If not, a member of the administration staff offered an appointment as quickly as possible. Also, on occasions a person would seek help or be referred urgently on the basis that a spouse or partner insisted they do so, because the trauma in the life of the primary sufferer was having such an adverse impact on family and their marital relationship.

One in ten patients were referred to other services. Referral to other specialisms or routine primary or community services was considered to be an important feature of the Centre's work. Sometimes this was a direct transfer because it was deemed that the person's needs should be addressed by another service, without any expectation of the person being referred back to the Centre. Sometimes, following assessment at the Centre, the person would be referred back to their family doctor or consultant for a medication review, prior to or alongside the commencement of trauma-focused therapy. On other occasions the referral related to specific problems and usually in this situation the Centre staff would take on a case management role to ensure the person got access to the service they had been referred for and to put in place arrangements for them to come back to the Centre or simultaneously to proceed with therapy in the Centre. Sometimes this case management function was undertaken by another agency – in agreement with the Centre. The case management function was important because it was concluded that many people suffering trauma-related problems after an initial sense of urgency about seeking help, might withdraw from help-seeking and engaging in services – particularly if it seemed that there were too many obstacles in the way.

The therapy programme – some considerations

Therapy would commence as soon as practicable following the assessment. This was usually rapid but sometimes, due to demands on the therapists and other work commitments within the Centre, some patients would have to wait some weeks before their therapy commenced. The randomised controlled trial undertaken by the Centre in 2005–2006 revealed that patients who concluded their therapy had an average of just over nine therapy sessions (Duffy et al., 2007).

The therapy programme typically involved regular attendance by patients at the Centre in Omagh. As noted already, routinely, standardised assessment tools were used to support the initial assessment and to enable patients and therapists to track progress session by session. Patients were asked to come 15 minutes prior to their appointment and to complete the instruments, which were then used in the therapy session. Patients responded well to the instruments and welcomed the objective feedback they illustrated on their progress. Where, exceptionally, a patient preferred not to use them or where the patient had literacy limitations, alternative approaches were used.

The developing clinical experience and the Centre's research led to the conclusion that trauma-related experiences and disorders are, for many patients, one of the key problems, if not the central problem, in their lives. This then has consequences in many aspects of their health, relationships and social and economic functioning. The Centre's work and research pointed to the place of cognitions and loss in such consequences, where for example traumatic experiences had adversely shaped the person's view of themselves, others and the world with further adverse implications for attachments and identity. 'I am not the person I used to be, or thought I was,' being a common post-trauma appraisal.

Building upon Ehlers and Clark (2000), the work of the therapy team at the Centre reinforced the benefits of systematically addressing patients' memory problems, the unhelpful appraisals they had developed of themselves, of others or of the world in general, and the unhelpful things they did or ways of thinking they used to manage the distress associated with the traumatic experience. Therapists typically employed curiosity and experimentation (where patients tested out revised perceptions of their inner and outer worlds); homework (where, for example, at an appropriate time in therapy, progress was tested out in the person's everyday world); activity, thought and mood monitoring in an effort to pinpoint triggers, thinking patterns and styles of the patient's way of viewing, thinking about, responding emotionally to or behaving in their world (Duffy, 2014; Duffy and Gillespie 2009).

One further consideration had become apparent through the work in the original Community Trauma and Recovery Team. It was noted that people suffering PTSD often presented with additional mental health and related problems, such as depression, other anxiety disorders or drug or alcohol dependency. This was particularly so the longer the time from the traumatic experience (or the onset of PTSD-related symptoms) until the point people sought assistance. Indeed it was usual for those who had PTSD for longer than six months to also have one or more recognisable mental health disorder.

One question that arises from this is whether PTSD is a precursor to the onset of additional disorders, or whether the prior existence of other disorders – such as depression – somehow precipitate PTSD. Therapists at the original Omagh Team and the new Centre observed that focusing on and addressing PTSD or groups of trauma symptoms seemed to be the key to addressing a range of problems experienced by patients. Very often reductions in trauma symptoms to below clinical levels were accompanied by considerable improvements in other problems including depression, other anxiety disorders and alcohol dependency for example. The reasons are perhaps more complex than this observation suggests. Ahead of, or alongside their intervention for PTSD, and based on a formulation of the person's needs and therapeutic priorities, therapists would address mental health problems other than PTSD. Also, where other problems or risks seemed to be a more immediate clinical or patient priority, this was addressed first. Referral to other services occurred commonly where, for example, alcohol dependency featured as the dominant and primary problem or where a physical health problem was the primary concern.

The first report on the wider population impact of the conflict by the Centre, as part of the NICTT-UU research partnership, cast some more light on the co-occurrence of PTSD and other disorders. One of the questions investigated was how depression relates to PTSD. The study showed that:

- of those who met the criteria for both depression and PTSD, 39% met the criteria for depression before the traumatic experience associated with their PTSD.
- 43.5% met the criteria for depression simultaneously to the onset of PTSD symptoms (1.6% met the criteria from the time of the traumatic experience but before the onset of PTSD).
- 21.7% met these criteria after the onset of PTSD. (Ferry et al., 2008).

On a note of caution, some of those who met the criteria for depression following their traumatic experience might have acquired depression for reasons not related to their traumatic experience or their PTSD. However, the findings reinforced the observations from practice that disorders found in association with PTSD often arise as a result of the traumatic experience or the struggle with PTSD, and often greatly improve when the PTSD is treated.

The Centre's therapy programme in the context of conflict

As the Centre was commencing its work in 2002, the years of violence were giving way to a peace process and a developing primacy of democratic politics. Whilst political agreements were in place to better manage the conflict, its legacy remained an issue of debate and division. Deep memories of the years of violence still existed, with many unresolved issues relating to them and their consequences, feelings of unaddressed and unresolved injustices, and non-state armed groups still using violence. Also, not everyone agreed with the political and peace processes.

Working in the context of civil conflict posed considerable challenges, which were of greatest importance to patients and staff, not least as getting things wrong could have had very serious implications. At a practical level, the Centre was open to seeing people from across the political-cultural spectrum, including civilians, people involved in public roles, or in emergency services. The management of appointments was important. For example, some patients had deep anxieties especially at early stages of their engagement with the Centre. Appointments were arranged at times which best suited patients. Safety was another consideration, especially for those who believed they were under a death threat. A third potential consideration was the need to be aware of arranging appointments so that patients from different experiences of the conflict, and who might be concerned at meeting each other, did not meet when they attended the Centre.

The Centre had adopted the position of being open to anyone who felt they could benefit from its services. This meant the Centre was acceptable to some but unacceptable to others. Some in the latter group would have preferred to access a service identified with their own cultural identity, or provided by an organisation associated with the groups of victims and survivors of the conflict they identified with.

The Centre's openness to engage with people who had different backgrounds and experiences gave rise to discussions amongst the clinical and management team on the function of a trauma service in the context of a civil conflict. The therapy team concluded that the therapeutic task required therapists to focus on the experiences that gave rise to trauma-related problems and associated difficulties, and on the therapeutic goals they and the patient had identified.

There was also the issue of where the Centre stood more generally on violence, specifically violence as an instrumental political means of bringing about change, or in securing the status quo. In practice, when focusing on the here-and-now needs of individuals, this was not a major issue. It did mean that in the context of

Northern Ireland the Centre took the view that the instrumental use of violence could not be endorsed. This was central to the core principles and origins of the Centre. Indeed it would have been very difficult to take an alternative view whilst offering a service aimed at addressing the consequences of violence. Whilst working in other countries affected by war and conflict where the sectarian lines and experiences of violence were even more starkly drawn than in Northern Ireland, Centre staff were aware that mental health practitioners sometimes strongly identified with the community they were serving (usually their own community). This presented itself in deep feelings about 'the enemy' and their violence, and the necessity of violence in addressing the violence of the enemy. Also, some practitioners in other contexts of war and conflict, including some who visited the Centre, spoke of their difficulty in understanding the position taken by the Centre on this matter, and at times were very uncomfortable with it.

The legal definition of victims and survivors in Northern Ireland gave rise to discussions about the role of the Centre and more widely the therapeutic function, in the context of civil conflict. During the time the Centre was operating the definition was determined by legislation passed in 2006 to be:

Article 3 – paragraph 1
(a) someone who is or has been physically or psychologically injured as a result of or in consequence of a conflict-related incident;
(b) someone who provides a substantial amount of care on a regular basis for an individual mentioned in paragraph (a); or
(c) someone who has been bereaved as a result of or in consequence of a conflict-related incident.
And [paragraph] (2) Without prejudice to the generality of paragraph (1), an individual may be psychologically injured as a result of or in consequence of (a) witnessing a conflict-related incident or the consequences of such an incident; or (b) providing medical or other emergency assistance to an individual in connection with a conflict-related incident. (Para 3; Victims and Survivors (Northern Ireland) Order, 2006).

This was sufficiently inclusive to not pose any significant problems for the Centre, although occasionally someone would approach the Centre for help who, it could have been argued, did not fit the criteria. The Centre staff took the widest possible view on the basis that if somebody needed help whose life had been adversely affected by their experiences of violence, then they should receive it. This could have been an issue if funders, particularly governmental funders, took a very strict legal view of who was entitled to services it funded for victims, survivors and carers.

Centre staff had conversations with politicians and others about the definition of victims and survivors for the purposes of accessing services, which included discussing the implications of narrowing the definition to exclude certain groups. One question for example, was whether people who were injured in carrying out an illegal act of violence should be entitled to services. Such questions give rise to a number of ethical and practical questions. The Centre took the view that to deny access on the basis of views about the nature of the help seeker's involvement in violence was fraught with a number of problems. First, as discussed above, different groups within the community took very different views as to the causes and legitimacy of the actions involving violence by members of non-state armed groups, the police or military. Second, limiting access to services might run foul of equality and disability legislation, and more widely, human rights provisions. More pragmatically, the Team argued that if someone had reached a point where they sought help then the proper response was to provide them with appropriate services. This was an ethical-moral issue. The same argument would apply to people seriously physically injured who required emergency or other hospital services. Could a civilised society expect or call upon medical and nursing staff to refuse to treat someone, for example, who had been injured in carrying out an act of violence, even one which led to the death and injury of others? And who would arbitrate such matters? (Other examples might include someone who causes a road collision in which others are injured or killed. Or someone whose lifestyle damages his or her health and who needs access to publicly funded health services.) It was also realised that it was not always easy to draw a line between perpetrators and victims. Some who were responsible for acts of violence might also have been victims of violence. Sometimes the experience of being a victim (for example, having someone close to you killed) might be the motivation for getting involved in armed groups or becoming a soldier or police officer, all of which might have involved the use of violence. If such a person was a member of an illegal organisation or responsible for illegal acts of violence, should they be excluded from therapeutic services if they had needs relating to their earlier experiences of being a victim of violence? Conversely, some who had been involved in acts of violence might subsequently have been a victim of violence – in association with or separate from their violent actions. Should they also be excluded?

The Centre took the view that they should be included if referred. It was thought that efforts to help people live constructively with their past actions and experiences, and make a more positive contribution to the future as a consequence of overcoming psychological distress and mental health disorders, was the appropriate response. This approach was part of the wider task of the caring professions acting in the interests of all citizens, as an ethical or moral response, and as the appropriate response, to the needs they had identified. Also, the Centre was part of the necessary response to the public health impact of the years of violence, and the contribution of therapeutic services was part of the wider task of making and securing peace. The approach was also in line with the trustees' ambition that the Centre would contribute to the transformation of individuals and society.

Therapy protocols

The Centre continually documented its therapy protocols, which had been developed initially in the original Omagh Community Trauma and Recovery Team. It was thought that the protocol could be finalised into a finished product, but it never was. For reasons to do with the on-going learning from the work of the Centre, the experiences of patients, messages from research, the specific requirements of funders, and issues relating to the post-conflict context of the work, the protocol seemed to be always changing. In the end it was decided that this could and probably should never be a finished product but a living one that would be constantly changed and updated. Nevertheless, having a written protocol was a very useful tool for the induction of new staff and as a reference against which practice could be evaluated. The protocol included referral criteria, arrangements for screening, assessment and therapy, risk management, matters relating to medication, data capture requirements, and recordings of therapy sessions. As each version was developed, the date of implementation was noted on the new rendition for ease of reference, and so reviews of patients at any point could be undertaken with reference to the relevant version of the protocol (NICTT, 2003).

Early interventions after traumatic experiences

At an early stage in the life of the Centre it was approached to provide services to people who had been involved in very recent traumatic events. This included traffic collisions, workplace accidents including farm accidents, house fires and events linked to the Troubles. The Centre had not expected to provide this service as it was focusing on people with longer-term trauma-related disorders. Also, being aware of controversies about early interventions after traumatic experiences, the clinical team was reluctant to offer an intervention when there were some uncertainties as to its effectiveness (e.g. Roberts et al., 2009). Yet the Centre was regularly asked to respond to such requests and as a Centre specialising in trauma-related needs it was difficult to argue that it had nothing to offer. To address this issue, members of the clinical team explored options for delivering an early intervention response. The literature was reviewed including the guidance of NICE (2005). The Centre's trauma therapy model was interrogated with the question, 'If we know what the components and mechanisms of trauma-related disorders are, what does this tell us about what we might do earlier to provide a meaningful intervention?' Out of this work, a psycho-educational intervention for people who had had recent traumatic experiences was developed and a protocol prepared (McLaren and Bolton, 2003). This, and subsequent updates, were used to guide interventions for recent traumatic experiences and to guide the Centre staff in supporting, reviewing and referring people who were seen within this sub-programme. The therapeutic service for people who had recently experienced a traumatic event was in keeping with the 'watchful waiting' recommended by NICE (2005). In summary, minimal information was obtained about the traumatic event – building up more detail in subsequent sessions. Trauma-related appraisals by the person of themselves, others or their wider world were noted but not interrogated (except to secure a clear understanding of what was being said). Information was also sought about the lifestyle and self-care of the person. Guidance was provided in relation to the benefits of social support, the disadvantages of isolating oneself, the importance of the maintenance of routine, sleep, diet and exercise, the adverse impact of reliance upon alcohol, street or prescribed drugs, and other areas. Sometimes partners chose to attend with the person who was seeking help or had been referred, and their input was most often valuable in identifying problems, in providing explanations and guidance, in reinforcing beneficial responses and later recalling the conclusions of the consultation. The subtext was an expectation of adjustment and recovery, which, if it seemed necessary or helpful to do so, was explicitly expressed. In the event of problems persisting or getting worse or of other problems being identified, access to therapy or help in accessing other services was offered. Finally, reviews over one to two months were offered and agreed with the therapist until such times as the person felt they were much better – or needed access to other services.

The service was not subjected to formal evaluation but anecdotally it was concluded that at the very least it offered reassurance at a time of deep distress or concern and supported families in coping with a difficult time. Feedback from patients suggested that the information and guidance provided was practical, relevant and generally well received, as was the expectation of coping and recovery and the availability of services if this did not occur.

Managing the therapy programme

In the early years, the therapy programme was managed by the Centre's therapy team leader who coordinated the allocation of the referrals. With the clinical director he decided upon how assessments would be undertaken, which members of the therapy team would carry them out, and the allocation of assessed patients to the therapy programme. As part of this work the Team leader was also responsible for the maintenance of records, including paper-based records, information held on computers, and audio and video recordings of patient therapy sessions. In later years, the patient services liaison social worker facilitated enquiries, undertook initial assessments, and supported the work of therapists with individuals. Weekly supervision with the clinical director involved the full team of therapists, backed up by supervision with individual therapists. The Centre had supervisory support from the Centre for Anxiety Disorders and Trauma at the Institute of Psychiatry, Maudsley Hospital, King's College London which proved to be particularly relevant and helpful in addressing the complex needs of some patients. This external point of reference was important in helping the Centre to maintain its practice, to keep up with developments in the therapeutic and trauma field and to allow the work of the Centre to inform wider developments in policy and services in Northern Ireland, in response to the needs of those adversely affected by the Troubles.

The administration staff played a central role in taking information from referrers and ensuring that those seeking help, along with the information received about their needs, were drawn to the attention of the therapy team. They also maintained the paper and computer-based records relating to patients and the general administrative work of the therapy programme. As often as possible, a member of the therapy team was available to answer queries, meet those who called at the Centre and occasionally deal with urgent therapy-related matters. Liaison was maintained with key organisations and individuals who referred people to the Centre. For example, contact was maintained with local mental health services, family doctors, and victim and survivor organisations.

Confidence, trust and safety

It was clear that engagement with patients needed pathways in and out of therapy and that it was insufficient to think of providing a limited protocol-driven intervention. One of the key symptom groups of trauma-related disorders is avoidance and numbing. The avoidance of things, places, people, sensory experiences and artefacts that the person associates with the traumatic experience and related distress, often extends into the prospect of seeking help or engaging in therapeutic conversations about their distress. This anxiety about seeking help can be driven by thoughts such as 'Nobody will be able to understand my experiences, needs, reactions or distress'; or, 'If I begin to talk about this then it will be so distressing for me I will not be able to manage or survive'; or a sense of shame, guilt or low self-esteem about some aspect of the traumatic experience or how the person feels they have been coping since it happened.

In some situations, this took the form of deep suspicions about intentions of health or counselling services in general, or the Centre's therapy programme itself. The therapy team often observed these fears about seeking and engaging in help. Some patients felt that they could not impose upon the therapist the awfulness of their experiences. Particularly in the early therapy sessions, patients required assurances that they would not 'fall apart' by talking about their experiences, or that the therapist was capable of handling what was for them devastating experiences. To enable a working relationship to be established with the person seeking help, it was important for the therapist to convey confidence in the ability to hear and to listen to the person's experiences and their consequences and to be able competently to handle the distressing content and emotional vulnerability. A supportive culture and supervision were key to supporting staff in managing what could be very distressing content in their work with patients.

In the context of the discord in Northern Ireland, such subjective senses of fear were often amplified by realistic or exaggerated concerns about personal safety as a result of general worries about being susceptible to acts of violence. Occasionally, enquirers or patients would explore or test out their anxieties about the Centre's position on their cultural identity, role or acceptability, before or during therapy, especially if some external event, such as news of a shooting or bombing, increased their sense of anxiety.

Whilst the levels and forms of violence had dramatically reduced since the ceasefires of the early and mid-1990s, for some the violence had not really ended. Armed groups which rejected the peace process and the new politics continued to be active and carry out acts of violence. Some exercised control within neighbourhoods, engaged in criminality or inter-group and inter-personal rivalries, sometimes with the use of violence. The Omagh bombing itself had been carried out by groups that had not embraced the political changes and agreements. For these reasons some people attending the Centre for therapy considered themselves to be under threat – either as a rational and understandable anxiety or more vividly, because they had been told they were under threat from one armed group or another, or they had personally received such death threats. Sadly, sometimes such death threats led to people dropping out of their engagement with therapy, in which case efforts were made to ensure they had other forms of support until, hopefully, they felt able to re-engage. Attacks on other people not related to the Centre nor perhaps even known to patients, also had an adverse impact on occasions, although it could also result in people seeking help for the first time. On one occasion a policeman was killed within a kilometre of the Centre after a bomb under his car exploded. His death was particularly distressing for some and resulted in patients withdrawing from therapy. Others refocused their therapy goals. Some with long-standing trauma problems approached the Centre for the first time, because the murder had caused them to examine their own coping strategies and need for assistance with long-term problems. For such reasons, establishing and building confidence of prospective or current patients was essential. Sometimes considerable preparatory work was required to enable people to engage in therapy, to agree what the therapeutic goals should be, and to remain engaged. As a result of specific death threats the immediate stressful circumstances were given priority, and therapy goals reviewed and refocused to address changing circumstances.

The distinctive challenges just described are an extension of the need for the therapist (and the agency) to establish a working therapeutic relationship with the person seeking help, and – if they engage – with them as a service user. Building and establishing trust is essential. The simple human values of welcome, warmth and respect are essential features of the therapist's, and his or her organisation's, engagement with the person seeking help. Against the background of civil conflict, safety is also a consideration, although this could not be guaranteed fully. The Centre was reluctant to put in place visible safety apparatus or arrangements that would themselves inhibit some individuals or groups of potential service users or that would draw attention to the Centre. Flexibility on the part of the therapist, plus the willingness to support the patient in shaping their own therapeutic goals and in revealing their deepest fears, shame or guilt, are also vital components of the therapeutic relationship. And, even in the face of such darkness, the use of humour – respectful humour – by the patient and the therapist has its place, for example, in permitting the safe observation of feelings, thoughts and experiences or as a way of finding new metaphors through which the person can be enabled on their therapeutic journey.

The isolation caused by trauma and its consequences

Earlier it was noted how isolated those who have suffered psychological problems linked to traumatic experiences can feel. This seemed to derive in part from the fundamental existential transformation traumatic events have on how people view themselves, other people or the world in general as a consequence of their experiences (Janoff-Bulman, 1985). Sometimes people just could not comprehend or make sense of what they had experienced, how they were reacting, or their new views and outlooks – often laden with dark and negative sentiments. It was not uncommon to hear patients report that they thought they were going mad, or that they were the only person in the world who felt the way they felt. As a consequence, some thought that their needs could never be understood and that they were beyond help. This fatalistic and deeply isolated place led to anxieties and a sense of stigma about seeking help. People struggled through, pretending there was nothing wrong, never disclosing, or sometimes to just a few, their extreme inner distress. Some spoke of how they 'wore masks', went through life 'like a robot' or 'made a brave face of it', which allowed them to get through the day or to hide their inner turmoil and distress from others. In such situations, sometimes it was a catastrophic mental or physical collapse, or key life events (e.g. an illness, birth of a child, retirement) that led to the person being referred.

Re-claiming valued and lost aspects of life

Many people adversely affected by traumatic events, especially over many years, cease partaking in interests and activities that they previously enjoyed. Sometimes they may never commence new interests even though life creates opportunities for them to do so, for example, after their children grow up and leave home, or after retirement. When it became clear after a period of progress in therapy that further steps might be taken, then thinking about resuming abandoned pleasures and pastimes was sometimes one of the options discussed by the therapist with the patient. Small achievable challenges were constructed as part of the therapeutic process, to test out the new preliminary or revised view of the person themselves, other people or the world in general. Judging the timing and the preparation for such steps was very important as negative outcomes could be a setback for patients. When successfully completed, the impact on patient confidence and morale was usually striking, encouraging further progress and experimentation.

Sometimes patients were so demotivated or demoralised by their experiences or traumatic events and their consequences that they needed some support before engaging in the therapy itself. The Centre's patient services liaison social worker, usually with the guidance of a therapist or the clinical director, would engage with the patient to help them reclaim aspects of their lives. This was with a view to, for example, lifting their mood and motivation to the point where they were more likely to engage with and benefit from therapy. In a number of cases, this had unanticipated favourable outcomes for those initially assessed as suffering with chronic PTSD to the extent that patients' trauma-related symptoms were found to be below clinical levels at the end of this grounding phase. One explanation is that, in the safe environment of therapeutic support, the resumption of abandoned sources of enjoyment and fulfillment or valued relationships, activities or pastimes, enabled and reinforced setting aside efforts to keep the trauma at a distance (i.e. avoidance). This resulted in the person beginning to process the traumatic experience, possibly for the first time, knowing they had the support of the therapy team. By engaging with the traumatic experience and its consequences, patients did what most do soon after a traumatic experience, that is, they began to process the experience. By the time they were ready to begin trauma-focused therapy, trauma-related symptoms had dramatically improved – much beyond what might have been anticipated. Further research into this could help gain a better understanding of the processes involved and possibly assist in identifying those who are likely to benefit from this type of intervention. As a consequence, those who need access to trauma-focused therapies as normally recommended for chronic PTSD could be more readily identified and prioritised.

Evaluating therapy in the context of conflict

Routinely, therapists evaluated each therapy session and a programme of therapy, aided by the standardised instruments used in the Centre. The therapy team engaged in supervision and work management on an almost weekly basis. Also, the Centre continued to have access to support from external links it had established in Northern Ireland, England and the United States of America, through which it sought advice, access to additional services, or help with the management of therapy for individual patients.

The Centre's work also offered the possibility of undertaking more formal research to assess how effective trauma-focused CBT was in addressing the distinctive, intense and complex therapeutic needs of patients living in a conflict and post-conflict context.

It was clear from the earlier work of the Community Trauma and Recovery Team that the Centre would be able to do this. During the first twelve months following the Omagh bombing, the town was subjected to 80 or more bomb alerts; these took the form of anonymous warnings by telephone to the police or other agencies, of a bomb having been placed in the town, which often resulted in significant disruption and evacuating part of the town. Such events had immediate distressing consequences for many patients attending the Centre's predecessor, the Omagh Community Trauma and Recovery Team. As described earlier, the original Omagh Team recognised that it was important to attend to these dynamic circumstances which patients found themselves in. This led to the reviewing and changing of therapeutic goals with patients. Ironically, it was learned that these adverse circumstances could be turned to advantage to help patients see that unhelpful cognitions and views of oneself, others or the world were most usually not universal. For example, through the experience of the bomb scares a person could be helped to see that their trauma-related fear – that they would never be able to cope at such times – was based on an inaccurate or incomplete view or appraisal of themselves, others and the world. This was especially so where, with the help of a therapist, they found in fact they could cope with and survive the most feared of circumstances.

After the Centre had been operational for a number of years, a report was provided by the NICTT to the Omagh Fund on an audit of therapy outcomes for those who had been referred to the Centre and who had been adversely affected by their experiences of the Omagh bombing. At the time of the report, forty-six had been referred, of which fourteen had completed the trauma-focused CBT programme provided at the Centre. The remainder were awaiting assessment, were engaged in therapy, or had not followed through with therapy after assessment. An audit of therapy outcomes for those who had completed therapy and had been discharged showed marked reductions in trauma and depression scores. The mean scores for trauma and depression at assessment were 32 (BDI) and 28 (PDS) – both significantly high measures. At discharge, the scores were 12 (BDI) and 6.5 (PDS), illustrating marked reductions in the symptoms for both conditions. (Kerr et al., 2006).

Soon after the Centre opened, planning began for a randomised controlled trial to assess the effectiveness of trauma-focused CBT for people with PTSD and related disorders as a consequence of the Troubles. This study was undertaken during 2003–2006 and was the subject of a paper published in 2007 (Duffy et al., 2007). The study is described in more detail in Chapters 5 and 9. The discipline of undertaking the study contributed to the systems and arrangements within the Centre for the therapy programme and the maintenance of records. When the study was completed these arrangements largely remained in place.

The patient group who took part in the study were typical of the wider group of the 670 or so who were referred to the Centre between 2002 and 2011. The primary data from the study is important as an illustration of the human experiences and consequences of the conflict in Northern Ireland. The picture revealed by the data is of relevance to politicians, policy-makers, service commissioners and providers, and practitioners in communities that have suffered enduring periods of violent civil discord. The experience of the study demonstrated the value of taking a research-based approach to the delivery of therapy services. Also, patients generally welcomed the fact that they were taking part in a study or that the Centre had a research programme through which the therapy they and others were receiving was continually being evaluated and developed.

Emerging needs and hidden victims

Both local and international epidemiological research showed that whereas males are more likely to be exposed to traumatic events, when females are exposed to them, they are more likely to develop PTSD (Bunting et al., 2013). The Centre's therapists saw approximately equal proportions of males and females, though in the latter years, more males. This pattern most probably reflected the much higher number of males who were exposed to the violence of the Troubles. Although, it is important to register that when men suffer the consequences of exposure to conflict-related violence, many women (mothers, wives, partners, sisters, daughters etc.) are left to pick up the pieces, to manage the impact on families, and suffer their own emotional, social and economic consequences.

It seemed that males were also seeking help much later than females, and not infrequently it was noted that men presented after many years of struggling with trauma-related disorders. Men seemed to have had relatively little contact with health or family doctor services, with even less contact in relation to their trauma needs. It was observed that men seemed to be referred to the Centre most often by their family doctors, through liaison staff working, for example, with ex-service personnel, or as a result of friends or colleagues having engaged with the Centre. The revelation of these hidden victims, who do not appear in the formal lists of casualties or the membership lists of victims' and survivors' organisations, became an increasingly important consideration in addressing the enduring impact of the Troubles.

Other factors influenced the levels of referrals. As political progress was made and the anxieties about large-scale violence decreased during the years the Centre was operating, more people who had previously somehow managed or lived with their distress came forward for help. There seemed to be a number of reasons why people sought help later. Partly it related to the failure or destructiveness of coping strategies that might have seemed to help initially. For example, social withdrawal, working very hard to keep the inner distress under control or becoming increasingly dependent upon alcohol. With political progress and the reductions in violence, it appeared that for many who were locked in their experiences of the violence, the world was cynically moving on. The optimism of peace, and the distancing from the years of violence which many in the community were experiencing, dramatically changed the situation for people suffering mental health problems who had coped up to the point of seeking help. With progress came the erosion of solidarity, as old community and segregation-based certainties yielded to a new, if uncertain, set of world views. It was common to hear patients ask, in relation to their experiences of the Troubles, or their commitment to various roles in the context of the Troubles, 'What was it all for?' It was clear too that some who had suffered violence felt that in moving on, the wider community had all too easily forgotten their personal suffering or losses. The loss of friends or colleagues through old age and death, or because they had moved away to live elsewhere, seemed another factor. Erosion or realignment of former identities and allegiances, and disillusionment with the perceived abandonment of political principles and objectives in furtherance of a political settlement, were a further cause of disconnection. These losses of the ideological and emotional structures of solidarity seemed to precipitate crises in the lives of people who had otherwise coped up to that point. These crises led them to seek help.

Conclusions

At the time the Centre's dedicated trauma-focused therapy programme was established, it was unique in Northern Ireland. The momentum for the development of the therapy programme provided by the Centre had been driven by a number of factors. These included the fact that a trauma-focused therapeutic service, which had already been tried and tested following the Omagh bombing, had proven to be highly relevant to a wider population affected by the Troubles. There was, therefore, a core of experienced practitioners available to form a therapeutic team. The pattern of demand from the public and the experience of the Centre demonstrated the need for open access specialist trauma-focused therapy services. Evidence of late help-seeking, from both the Centre's therapy and research programmes, suggested that after years of violent conflict these services would be required for some time to come. To fill the evident lack of routinely accessible specialist services, the Centre's work revealed that here was a clear need for new and continuing investments in specialist and auxiliary trauma-focused services, to play their part alongside other health and supportive services and initiatives.

8

Trauma-focused skills training for practitioners

This chapter describes the Northern Ireland Centre for Trauma and Transformation (NICTT)'s training development and delivery programmes over ten years, focusing in particular on vocational training. The aim was to build the skills base of existing practitioners by providing a number of cognitive behavioural therapy (CBT) and trauma-related skills courses. The approach taken was to build courses which addressed the needs of service users, and to develop the skills required by practitioners to do this.

Background

The Centre's trustees and staff saw training, education and specifically skills development as an important aspect of its work. This was reflected early on in the Centre's mission statement, to 'Treat trauma, advance learning and contribute to transformation'. The training and education work had an advocacy function in that it was aimed at increasing knowledge of the needs and service requirements of those adversely affected by their experiences of the violence in Northern Ireland (see Chapter 9). The intention was also to support the development of skills for working effectively with patients and clients and especially to raise knowledge, skills and capability concerning trauma-related needs. It was most helpful that the evidence base supporting CBT approaches to trauma-related needs was quite well established when the Centre opened. Within two years, Northern Ireland's health department published guidance on the management of PTSD in adults (DHSSPS, 2003). Two years later, in England, the National Institute for Health and Care Excellence published guidance on the management of PTSD in children and adults (NICE, 2005). The Centre was open to the development of other approaches to trauma-related needs should the opportunity arise and funding become available. For example, a number of therapists had been trained in EMDR (Eye Movement Desensitisation and Reprocessing) which, along with trauma-focused CBT, had been recommended in the DHSSPS and NICE guidance for the treatment of PTSD.

Early training developments

Training delivered by the Centre early on built upon previous work by the clinical director, who had developed and delivered a programme of CBT skills-focused short courses. Within three years of opening, the Centre had delivered a four-day skills based course to 240 health and social care practitioners and service managers working mainly in the public sector. This was funded through the European Union's Interreg IIIA and Peace II programmes and involved practitioners from Northern Ireland and the border counties of the Republic of Ireland. The training pointed the way for further workforce development. Part of the ambition for the course was to build the interest in CBT, in the hope that at least some who took part would in time go on to take postgraduate diploma courses that would allow them to practice as CBT therapists. Later, through a partnership with the Belfast Trauma Advisory Panel – one of five such interagency panels that were established to assist with the coordination of service development and responses to people and communities affected by the years of violence – a postgraduate diploma and masters course on CBT, with a specialist module on the treatment of PTSD, was developed at Ulster University. This course was provided for four years.

The impact of international experiences

The experiences that staff from the Centre had in other countries affected by conflict played a key part in the thinking about how training could be developed. During a visit to Sarajevo in Bosnia in 2006, a training programme based on the Centre's work was delivered to mental health practitioners and therapists who were mainly working with people affected by the conflict in the Balkans and in particular the siege of Sarajevo and the impact of the war on Goražde (1991–1999). The needs being confronted by the Bosnian psychiatrists and therapists were severe and highly challenging from a therapeutic perspective. Earlier, a similar programme had been delivered in 2005 to mental health workers in Sri Lanka, who were dealing at that time with the legacy of the country's civil war and with the terrible consequences of the Indian Ocean tsunami of December 2004. These encounters with practitioners in areas affected by disaster and conflict were highly informative. The Centre's team had to construct short courses based on its work that could be delivered over a few days with the added requirement and obstacle of translation. The need to work across languages required a high level of precision and succinctness, as well as the avoidance of idioms and short cuts people often use when conversing with others in a common language. Much was gained from this work. Perhaps most of all, the confidence that it was possible to disassemble the otherwise coherent philosophy and practice of trauma-focused CBT into discrete areas of competence, which could then be taught, and make an impact, in highly demanding circumstances. The work also revealed how people have much in common across cultures in the face of human experiences of loss and trauma. Models of intervention relating to these common human experiences and needs, sensitive to forms of expression, cultural reference points, metaphors and ways of seeing the world, could be of assistance across and within cultures. One memorable occasion with a Buddhist community in Sri Lanka, desperately affected by the tsunami, involved their leader simultaneously translating and illustrating on a flip-chart what was being said for her colleagues – in a way that all could understand. Later the Centre, in conjunction with another non-governmental organisation based in Northern Ireland and a local one in Pokhara, Nepal, developed and delivered a two-year trauma-focused psycho-social programme aimed at raising knowledge and skills about trauma and other psycho-social needs, with particular relevance to the Maoist-military civil conflict in Nepal from 1996 to 2006 (Brown, 2009). This involved a social worker from Nepal spending four months at the Centre in Omagh, during which time she undertook the Certificate in Cognitive Therapy Methods (described below), prior to the commencement of the programme itself in Pokhara and the surrounding rural Districts.

The lessons from Northern Ireland and elsewhere

Through these international experiences and the work in Northern Ireland, it was realised that in areas of high need – with low levels of resources relative to that need – the ideal of training therapists to the optimum post-graduate masters level could never be accomplished fast enough, not least because there were insufficient trainers, supervisors and places on courses. Rather, the focus in such circumstances had to be on skilling-up existing practitioners who were already in contact with, or were close to, communities and individuals affected by war, conflict or disaster. It was also learned that as well as offering training to practitioners, their organisations needed to be enabled to understand, facilitate and incorporate the new skills once the training was completed. Otherwise the benefit of the training could be lost or minimised. As outlined above, these lessons were applied in the Nepali programme.

All this had echoes for the Centre's work in Northern Ireland. It was already clear from the research undertaken after the Omagh bombing by the original Omagh team, and the profile of people attending the Centre for therapy, that the needs were great in terms of severity and numbers. Some way had to be found to build up the capacity of existing services. This was at least as important an objective as the production of post-graduate therapists who would be capable of addressing the more complex needs of individuals. A similar developmental challenge applied to the provision of supervision for practitioners delivering trauma-focused therapy services.

These observations were borne out by the therapeutic work of the Centre's therapists. Patients attending the Centre commonly reported problems in reaching a point where they could seek help with trauma-related anxieties and problems – an inherent feature of trauma-related disorders, specifically PTSD (discussed in some detail in Chapter 7). They also reported, or it was clear from their histories, that their trauma-related needs had not been understood previously even though they had often had earlier contact with health or counselling services. Had their needs been identified and understood much sooner after their traumatic experience, and appropriate services offered, then many would probably not have required more specialist services later and the longer-term problems could have been avoided or minimised. People presenting early were generally much more likely to have less complex problems and would be helped more readily than those with longer standing problems.

As things stood in Northern Ireland there appeared to be insufficient awareness of, understanding of, or skills to deal with, trauma-related needs over and against the numbers of people with such problems. Access to trauma-aware services was not sufficiently and routinely accessible in a community where the levels of exposure to traumatic stress were significant. Also, the early skills raising programme revealed that practitioners and their managers welcomed training that renewed and sharpened forgotten practice principles and skills, or introduced them for the first time to principles and skills relevant to trauma and loss.

The need for a stepped-care trauma service

All this pointed to the need for an accessible, stepped and integrated trauma-focused approach. For example, when someone has a traumatic experience the known risks of developing psychological problems would be monitored. Thereafter, people presenting early with needs which are to one degree or another associated with traumatic experiences and their consequences would have an adequate assessment from which their difficulties would be better understood. The assessment would take account of the person's traumatic experiences and their wider health and life history and circumstances. Suitable primary and secondary level care services would be offered. This should include support from practitioners capable of understanding and working with trauma sufferers within their normal role – in community, primary, or secondary care services. Thereafter, if the person presented with more severe or chronic needs – or their earlier identified needs were not responding to community, primary or secondary interventions – they should be referred for specialist (third level or tertiary) services. Thereafter, people could be stepped down to less specialist services as their well-being improved or, if they had recovered, be discharged.

To achieve this, skills would need to be developed at all levels. At first-point-of-contact and in primary or first level services, the aim would be to develop

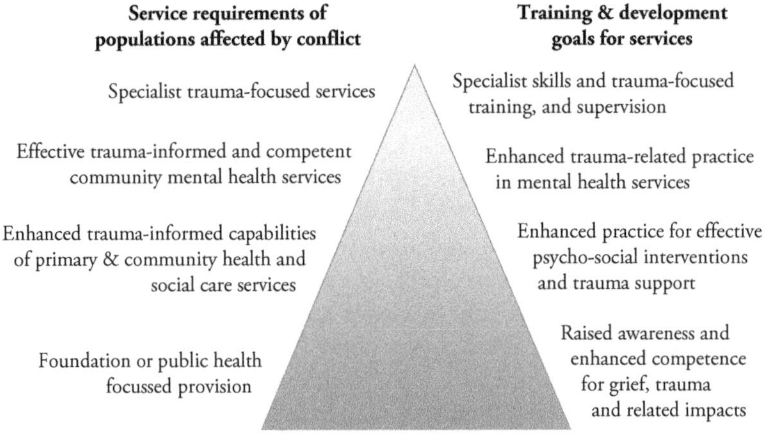
Service requirements of populations affected by conflict
Training & development goals for services
Specialist trauma-focused services
Specialist skills and trauma-focused training, and supervision
Effective trauma-informed and competent community mental health services
Enhanced trauma-related practice in mental health services
Enhanced trauma-informed capabilities of primary & community health and social care services
Enhanced practice for effective psycho-social interventions and trauma support
Foundation or public health focussed provision
Raised awareness and enhanced competence for grief, trauma and related impacts

Figure 5: A needs-led and trauma-focused public health framework for service development and building workforce capability in communities affected by long-term stressors.

competence in trauma awareness. This would ensure workers would have skills to identify and work with trauma, in their current roles. Thereafter, at specialist levels, the aim would be to ensure practitioners are trauma-focused, meaning they would be capable of bringing specialist trauma-focused skills to address severe trauma-related needs. The aim would be to develop coherent approaches whereby a common psychological orientation and literacy would inform the total service (Hannah and Leicester, 2006). Key to this was the development of an integrated skills based and trauma-related training framework that would be appropriate to the level practitioners were working at in relation to trauma. The need for this approach was promoted by the Centre at an early stage in its work. See Figure 5.

The Certificate in Cognitive Therapy Methods

Building on the early work, on the encouragement of the participants in the early courses, and on the experiences of preparing and delivering courses in international contexts, the Centre set about developing its integrated suite of courses. At the time, no off-the-shelf courses could be identified with the range of competences required by the Centre. The first course to be developed was its Certificate in Cognitive Therapy Methods (CCTM). This was achieved through the establishment of a partnership led by the Centre under the auspices of Cooperating and Working Together (CAWT) – a consortium of health and social care agencies on both sides of the Irish border, with funding from the European Union Interreg IIIA and Peace II programmes. The consortium involved health and social care commissioning agencies from Northern Ireland, the Western and Southern Health and Social Services Boards, the Republic of Ireland, and the border counties of the Health Service Executive West and Dublin North East regions. The EU funding also supported the development of a training-the-trainers programme and the earlier four-day skills based course discussed above (CAWT, 2008).

The Centre commenced the writing, accreditation and delivery of the 18-day course. It was decided that the course should be formally accredited. Instead of working with Universities where the main focus is on academic training, the Centre selected one of the UK's accrediting bodies (Edexcel) to develop and assign an appropriate vocational training level, to provide the professional oversight and to award the participants their certificates on successful completion. The course was written as a Certificate to Level 4 on the Qualifications and Credit Framework (QCF). The QCF is the national agency in England, Northern Ireland and Wales which oversees the arrangements whereby courses are assigned values in terms of vocational and academic levels and time.

How the course was written and developed

A needs-led approach was taken to the development of the course. This involved writing the course from scratch rather than using existing courses. The approach was taken after considering the experiences, needs and service requirements of patients and clients, and, second, the skills requirements of practitioners if they were to competently meet those needs. The planning also took account of experience and roles of the main body of practitioners in the publicly provided health system and in the not-for-profit sector. The thinking behind the course was that practitioners bring with them a wide range of experience, knowledge and skills particularly about systems and services. However, many of those who had taken part in the early preliminary programmes revealed that whilst they had been educated in certain theoretical approaches and trained in specific methods, they had not availed of more recent training in effective engagement with patients and clients since they were formally qualified as counsellors, health or social care practitioners. This was particularly important, as the course relied upon new ideas and methods based on research about working effectively with patients and clients. Many practitioners also indicated that their original pre-professional training had not addressed the health needs arising from the experiences of violence associated with the Troubles. The approach taken therefore considered what essential building blocks could be added to the existing experience, knowledge and skills of practitioners.

Over a number of intensive workshops lasting three to four days, the Centre's clinical director and director constructed the course and developed the competences which practitioners should be able to demonstrate in each area. The clinical director's experience in both practice and teaching in CBT was central to the selected areas that eventually made up the course and their contents. The course contents were made up of areas (units) that introduced CBT principles and skills to the students. The principles were considered to be of equal importance to the skills. With reference to the QCF, the learning outcomes for each unit were clearly defined, along with the evidence required to demonstrate that the student had successfully completed the unit. The experience of writing the course showed that it was tempting and in some senses easier to put too much content into it. It was soon clear that the amount of content initially identified would be unmanageable both for students and tutors. It was therefore through a process of continual refinement, fine-tuning and prioritisation that a core set of units and competences were identified, which were critical to the aims of the course. It was helpful for the writers to constantly remind themselves of the aims of the course (to address the needs of service users and to develop the skills of practitioners) and to likewise refer to the guidance issued by the QCF.

Meanwhile the Centre's business development manager identified suitable awarding bodies. When the training development team selected an accrediting body a formal application was made to have the course, and the Centre as training delivery agency, accredited. This required a business case to be written for the awarding body to demonstrate that there was sufficient economic demand for the course, and to demonstrate that the Centre had the capacity to deliver the training.

The response to the course

There was much interest in the course, which was delivered in locally accessible venues across Northern Ireland and the border counties of the Republic of Ireland. By the time the course ran for the last time, just before the Centre closed in 2011, several hundred practitioners from the public health and social care services and the not-for-profit sectors had participated – the vast majority of whom successfully completed the course. The fact that it was 'vocational' and not 'academic' did not prevent a wide range of health and social care practitioners, counsellors and others taking the course. The general view was that practitioners wanted ready access to quality training and the acquisition of relevant skills and knowledge. Other key advantages included the lower costs of the vocational training route for practitioners and their employers, and delivery by tutors who were simultaneously involved in providing therapy to people with psychological problems and mental health disorders. The delivery of the programme by specialist therapists brought credibility to the training and enabled real clinical issues raised by students to be explored in the context of the course.

Operations and service managers were very supportive of the course. They were required to give an assurance that the training was relevant to the work of their staff members. Also, that it was relevant to a client base whose needs were in one way or another linked to the Troubles. They were asked to provide an assurance that staff would be supported, both during the training and in the deployment of their new knowledge and skills once the course was ended. This support was enthusiastically offered and when managers saw how much their colleagues benefitted from the training they were often keen for other members of their teams to apply for places on the course.

For the first three courses, CAWT contributed funding which supported the development of the course, venues, travel and some staff replacement costs. The Centre's core training delivery costs were funded by Northern Ireland's health department, later by the Office of the Minister and Deputy First Minister, and other independent funders. The pump priming of training development needed both the additional funding to cover development and delivery costs (CAWT) and mainstream funding to support the core capability of the Centre.

The course had wider acknowledgement, and the Centre was awarded a National Training Award (Northern Ireland winner and UK finalist) in 2009 for it. At the time the Award was made, over two hundred practitioners working in the publicly provided and not-for-profit sectors had taken the course. In the citation from the awarding body, tribute was paid to the Centre's work in developing the training programme, and the fact that it had made a significant impact on health and social care practitioners and their patients and clients. The transferability of the course in international settings was also noted. As described earlier, in 2007 a social worker from Nepal had spent four months in Omagh studying with the Centre and had completed the training offered there. On returning to Nepal she then delivered a psycho-social programme and a counselling service for people affected by the civil conflict in Nepal.

Evaluation of the training

One of the most important sources of influence on specific courses and the overall training programme was the feedback from participants and their managers. Each CCTM course was closely evaluated. This included feedback from the daily interaction between tutors and participants, assessments by students of their baseline and end-of-course skills and knowledge, and independent evaluations undertaken by the awarding body, and in one case, a funder (Fee, 2008).

The baseline evaluation by students asked them to rate at the outset their own knowledge and skills on the range of subjects that were going to be covered in the course. Then, at the conclusion of the course they were asked to rate their knowledge and skill levels having completed the course. Finally they were asked to review the initial rating of their knowledge and skills (i.e. the assessment given prior to commencing the course). The ratings were recorded on questionnaires prepared by the Centre's team, which also allowed for additional free text comments from students. This approach revealed that participants usually overstated their assessment of their competences at the outset. When their end-of-course assessment was compared with their reviewed initial assessment, significant gains in their estimates of their knowledge and skills were revealed. An independent review of the baseline and end-of-course self-assessments by the first three groups of students (sixty in total) concluded 'there has been significant enhancement in the levels of cognitive therapy knowledge, skills and competence across all the learning outcomes during the period of attendance at these certificate programmes' (Fee, 2008: 14). Also, 'about a third of respondents reported they were concluding their work with patients/clients earlier since attending the course, with some respondents also reporting that they noted some reduction in the use of medication as a result of their work, using their new skills and learning' (p. 17).

This feedback was very useful in refining later courses of the CCTM. For example, it could be seen where the course was particularly successful and conversely, where students struggled more – hence the need for more time and input in the more challenging areas. Subsequent courses were modified or the areas where participants seemed to struggle more were addressed in refresher or master class workshops.

Even though the course had been designed specifically to address the locally determined needs of patients and clients and the skills and knowledge needed by practitioners to address those needs, Fee (2008) found that lack of supervision support in the workplace limited the capacity of staff who completed the course and their employers to deploy them optimally. This highlights the need for employers and service providers to make the most of training by putting in place arrangements to maximise the new learning and skill sets of students. This includes making provision for the deployment of the new skills, integrating the new skills into the wider work of the department or team and providing appropriate supervision and support.

In the more advanced training programmes that were subsequently developed by the NICTT, evaluation of skills gained was assessed by tutors using video recordings of therapy sessions, and marked against set criteria.

Further developments

By the time the Centre closed in 2011 it had developed the framework for an integrated trauma-related training programme. The programme involved five vocational courses, all of which were designed, written, accredited where possible and delivered by the Centre's team. The framework is summarised in Table 2. There were plans to add other relevant courses to this framework, either written by the Centre or acquired from courses already published on the UK's QCF.

Through the experience of developing the CCTM, the Centre contributed to the wider development of competences for CBT in the UK. That wider progress in the identification of national competences for a range of psychological therapies subsequently greatly assisted the development of the Centre's later and more advanced courses, in particular the Professional Diploma in Trauma-focused

Table 2: Overview of the NICTT's integrated trauma-focused workforce development framework

Course title	Length (days)	QCF level	Outputs
Introduction to Post Traumatic Stress Disorder	2	3	Delivered to approximately 300 practitioners
The Certificate in Cognitive Therapy Methods	18	4	Delivered to approximately 350 practitioners
Trauma-focused assessment and intervention for health and social care practitioners	2	4	An additional unit for the 18-day Certificate course – developed but not piloted
Professional Diploma in Trauma-focused Cognitive Behavioural Therapy	8	5	Piloted with one group of students
Advanced Professional Diploma in Supervisory Practice in Psychological Therapy	8	6	Piloted with one group of students

Cognitive Behavioural Therapy and the Advanced Professional Diploma in Supervisory Practice in Psychological Therapy (see Table 2).

The later courses were all written to specific QCF levels with a view to accreditation. All the experience gained in developing the CCTM was incorporated into the development of the later courses, including the structuring of course units, learning outcomes and evidence of skills or knowledge gained. The advanced courses were then piloted with groups of willing participants who provided feedback on the course, the design, the pace and the practice outcomes. Whilst these courses were developed and piloted by the Centre, due to its closure and the breakup of the training development team, they were not formally accredited with an awarding body nor made more widely available.

The implications of a trauma-focused approach

From the Centre's experiences of understanding training needs, developing, delivering and evaluating training courses a number of conclusions can be reached. First is the necessity of taking account of the specific needs of the population. This involved taking account of that part of the community's needs, represented by the Centre's patients, their carers and families (i.e. those who had been adversely affect in psychological, mental health and wider social terms by their experiences of the violence linked to the Troubles).

Second is taking account of the baseline of skills and competences of those who have an interest in trauma-focused training and in the services for which the training is intended. In the context of the Centre's work in Northern Ireland this involved recognising the interest of practitioners and service managers in, and their need for, new areas of knowledge and skills.

The years of violence had given rise to levels of trauma-related needs in the population of public health proportions (discussed further in Chapter 9). There was therefore much to be gained in taking a trauma-focused approach to thinking about service needs, workforce development and training. This brought a number of advantages. First, a trauma-focused approach mapped on to the presenting and core needs of the vast majority of patients seeking help from the Centre and other services. This then informed the way in which the Centre organised its services, including the representation of what it had to offer to potential service users and referring agencies.

Through a research-based explanatory model of trauma and how it could be addressed in the life of the individual (Ehlers and Clark, 2000) a trauma-focused approach also offered a way of understanding the experience and needs of the individual. In particular, the trauma-focused model used by the Centre identified the essential features of the adverse traumatic reaction – set in a theory of why we sometimes suffer adverse psychological traumatic responses to terrible life experiences. The model offered a way of understanding why we sometimes become traumatised, why those responses are maintained (instead of being resolved), what it takes for the person to address the need (including the struggle of asking for help), and therefore what the requirements and task of the trauma-focused therapeutic relationship are. The method helped to shape the total approach to the therapeutic task – mindful of the context of conflict – and allowed therapists to do the following.

- To enable and support the person's contemplation of seeking help and engagement (mindful of the inherent problems people suffering trauma-related disorders have in seeking help).
- To establish a sense of safety for the person seeking help (noting the additional challenges of doing this in the context of conflict when there was fear about safety or people were subject to actual death threats).
- To form a trusting and effective therapeutic relationship.
- To be able to use – and help the service user understand, engage with and deploy with support – the chosen approach or model.
- To undertake a trauma-aware assessment of the person's problems and history.
- To identify, agree on and continually revise the patient's therapeutic goals.
- To refer to other services where indicated.
- At more specialist levels, to address the traumatic experience(s) and consequences using the trauma-focused model, sometimes addressing various components simultaneously.
- At more specialist levels, to revise the narrative of the traumatic experience(s)

and consequences so that they are no longer a source of continuing distress but historical, if significant, life events.
- To end therapy with the person being aware of life problems overcome, aware of new skills and strengths, accepting of loses and limitations, engaged with prospects for the resumption of valued relationships, activities and preoccupations, and having confident expectations for further recovery and growth.

All of this had implications for training and development, as demonstrated above. The approach taken by the Centre provided a way of organising and determining the content of training, supervision and support needs of practitioners. Through its approach and experience, specific clues were gathered as to what levels of competence practitioners require to identify trauma-related issues and register the effect this is having within the person's life over and against other life challenges. It also clarified the benefits of establishing to what degree a traumatic event in the life of the person (including sustained periods of trauma exposure) was a driving or secondary issue in their life problems.

That led to thinking about what practitioners working in their everyday roles can do to support and assist people who have experienced traumatic events and are suffering adversely as a consequence; and to assist them with a degree of confidence, knowing when to refer their patients or clients for more specialist services. This was referred to as *the triage role* of workers who daily connect with trauma-affected populations. By triage, the Centre meant three things. First, the capability to recognise trauma-related problems. Second, the ability to work effectively within one's role and competence with a person who has trauma-related needs, and third, the ability to refer appropriately and in good time, to more specialised trauma-related services. Thereafter the Centre's approach and work also enabled clarity to be gained on what practitioners working at more specialist levels should be capable of achieving.

Having taken a trauma-focused approach the Team at the Centre was mindful of, and regularly reminded of, the need to be focused on trauma – but not to the exclusion of other ways of understanding the needs of individuals. As a specialist Centre, the therapeutic team was trauma-focused but not exclusively so. The trauma-focused approach was just the most important window on the needs of individuals. The work of the Team was set in the context of a wider body of knowledge of human need, in the daily experience of living in a community adversely affected by conflict, in knowledge of the impact of wider social, economic and environmental stressors and systems, and exemplified in the outward referral of one in ten of those referred to the Centre for other services.

Conclusions

These experiences and observations have implications for the way in which services for populations affected by violent conflict are organised and commissioned; also for the way in which training and development is approached and commissioned. The experience of the Centre suggests that commissioning for conflict-affected communities needs to be informed by evidence-based models of trauma and related needs. Knowledge about the scale and severity of needs should be at the heart of the modelling of service requirements, and thereafter, the resources, timeframe and funding needed to address the identified needs. The experiences of the Centre demonstrate the necessity of addressing trauma-related needs by service commissioners at the community and psycho-educational level, and at primary care, secondary and specialist levels. Workforce development and the requisite training needs to be commissioned in parallel with this service development so that skilled practitioners are increasingly available to populate the growing service provision. How all this is done should be informed by the experiences and views of those who need and access services and by the practitioners who endeavour to meet their needs. Finally, commissioners need be mindful of changing and trans-generational needs, again based on evidence, users' and practitioners' views, so that services are constantly being refined.

If there is an end to the task of meeting the needs of conflict-affected communities, then one aim is to ensure that in time – in spite of what the population has experienced – it is psychologically better off or healthier when the work is drawing to its conclusion. The legacy should be a better-equipped and informed public with more psychological know-how and skills, greater psychological resources at a personal and family level, with greater personal and collective resilience to face new difficulties. In terms of services, there would be sufficient appropriately trained and skilled practitioners, with commissioning and funding of services, and training, intelligently reflecting the changing needs of the post-conflict community.

9

Research, advocacy and policy support

This chapter considers the benefits of, and an approach to, undertaking research as part of the task of a trauma centre. Ongoing research into the changing needs of communities affected by emergency or conflict is fundamental to informing policy, advocating for service development, supporting the needs-directed commissioning of services and training, and to developing practice. Given limited resources – sometimes in the face of enormous needs – there are also key benefits in developing evidence of the effectiveness of supportive and therapeutic interventions for trauma-related and other disorders. The context of conflict throws up additional considerations and ethical questions for researchers.

The availability of evidence does not guarantee progress in policy, commissioning, service development, workforce development and practice. Systems responsible for delivering progress in these areas need to be both willing and able to use research data and conclusions to develop evidence-based responses. The use of the evidence in informing policy and service progress is discussed further below, along with some reflections on the factors that impact on progress.

Early efforts to understand needs after the Omagh bombing

As described earlier, it was the intention of those involved in forming and leading the response of the public health services, from the earliest hours and days following the Omagh bombing, that as much as possible should be learned from the tragedy in terms of impact, needs and service requirements. This aspiration and commitment was driven by the hope that the Omagh bombing would mark the end to violence once and for all, and that what could be determined would inform the response to the bombing itself, and offer the lessons learned for the wider benefit of those affected by the Troubles. Within the local public health and social care services provider there was therefore a strong commitment by both senior service managers and practitioners to understand and to learn as much as possible about the needs of those affected by the bombing, about their service requirements and about the delivery and effectiveness of therapeutic interventions and services. The efforts to understand and assess the impact of the bombing are described in Chapters 1, 2 and 3.

The level of data on the psychological and mental health impact of the bombing, most of which was being provided in 'near-real-time', was unique in the history of the Troubles. No previous tragedy associated with the Troubles had been the subject of such detailed investigation regarding the psychological impact, due largely to the political context of the bombing, the commitment of local agencies and the availability of well-tested tools by which the psychological and mental health impact could be assessed. This provided a unique and significant insight into the impact of major community tragedy, and from which potentially many valuable lessons could be learned – not just for the benefit of those affected by the bombing in Omagh – but for the wider benefit of those who suffered in psychological and mental health terms, from the Troubles.

Assessing needs and progress in therapy

The work of the Omagh Community Trauma and Recovery Team had highlighted the need to use well-tested tools (i.e. widely used research-based scales or questionnaires to assess psychological state and mental health disorders) for supporting assessments, therapy and for gathering information. It is important to use tools that have been tested for their ability to reflect as accurately as possible the needs and experiences of individuals (i.e. acuity). Such well-tested (or validated) tools allow the results to be compared with other national and international research-based means. It is important to have agreed practices and procedures in place for the use of the tools.

The practice that evolved in the Omagh Team was that one or more tools were completed at the outset of a person's assessment, usually at every therapy session thereafter, and at the conclusion of therapy. The changing needs and progress of patients were illustrated through this routine use of the tools. The picture they provided was of as much interest to the patients as they were to therapists, and they formed a very important part of the conversation between the patient and therapist. For example, if difficulties had increased during therapy – a common, if short-term occurrence as the trauma and its consequences were explored – then the tools often helped to focus on why problems had increased. This assisted the therapeutic process and collaboration between the patient and the therapist, helping to identify the driving thoughts behind the post-trauma reaction. Conversely, where the patient improved – as was generally the case – the scores tended to reinforce the experience of improvement, thereby reaffirming and encouraging the person in their adjustment and recovery.

Some practitioners and agencies had expressed anxieties about the use of such tools for those who sought help with trauma-related needs. The experience of the Omagh Team revealed, however, that when the purpose and benefits were explained to them, those seeking help were very content to routinely complete such tools as part of their therapy. One of the important effects was to underline the commonality of experiencing problems following traumatic events, and to helpfully challenge the thought that the person was alone in their distress and that their needs could not be understood. Patients were often profoundly reassured that their distress was not unique to them and that it was an experience of such commonality it had been incorporated into the instruments being used by the Team.

Apart from the immediate benefits for therapy, the information derived from the use of tools assisted in supervision, in the auditing of the therapy service and in building experience in how to develop research questions and procedures. Anonymised meta-data from groups of patients also provided very valuable material for ensuring that funders, politicians, political advisers, civil servants and others, were provided with information about the nature, severity of needs and the outcomes of therapy services. For example, it was the use of such data that enabled the Sperrin Lakeland Trust to make the case to the government for further funding to extend the life of the Omagh Community Trauma and Recovery Team from initial twelve months to two-and-a-half years. Amongst managers and practitioners, the early practice of capturing data about patient experiences, circumstances and needs, and about therapy processes and outcomes, helped to develop a culture of therapy-focused inquisitiveness, the desire to review, learn about and change methods and practice, and to contribute to wider learning through audit and research.

Research as a core programme of the NICTT

As the work of the Omagh Community Trauma and Recovery Team was drawing to a close (2000–2001), the proposals for what became the Northern Ireland Centre for Trauma and Transformation (NICTT) were being developed, and from an early stage included research and development as one of the key programmes. This was central to the profile of the Centre, not just because of the value of research itself. The relationships connecting therapy, the development and delivery of training, and research were interlocking. For example, what was learned through the therapy programme informed the research questions. The findings from research informed and influenced the therapy programme and the training and education work of the Centre. And so on. The merits of this interconnectivity amongst programmes was identified by Williams and Nurmi in their description of the archetypal comprehensive trauma centre which was discussed in Chapter 6 (Williams and Nurmi, 2001).

The NICTT randomised controlled trial

Once the NICTT therapy team was established, a research working group was formed to guide the development of the research programme. At an early stage it was decided that work should begin on a randomised controlled trial of the therapeutic approach (trauma-focused cognitive behavioural therapy (CBT)) being used at the Centre for the treatment of adults with trauma-related disorders. With the help of Professor David Clark and colleagues, then at the Institute of Psychiatry at King's College London, plans for the trial were developed in 2003–2004. The randomised controlled trial was subsequently undertaken, with fifty-eight consecutive patients who presented at the Centre and who met the criteria for PTSD; it was the subject of a paper published in 2007 (Duffy et al., 2007).

Foremost in the mind of the Centre's team was the aim of evaluating the effectiveness of a trauma-focused intervention for a population affected by political conflict, which had already been shown to be effective for PTSD in less turbulent circumstances. The study was designed, and ethical approval obtained. The Centre's therapy programme and treatment protocols were designed to reflect the requirements of the study. The Beck Depression Inventory (BDI) (Beck et al., 1988) and the Post-Traumatic Stress Diagnostic Scale (PDS) (Foa et al., 1997) were used to assess depression and trauma symptoms. Systems were put in place within the Centre to systematically capture data to a standard required by the study. When the trial commenced, additional mechanisms were put in place, such as arrangements for patient consent and the randomisation of patients to a waiting list or immediate access to therapy. Arrangements for supervision and various checks and balances to independently validate the assessment of patients were also established for the duration of the study. This approach meant that most of the costs of the study were accommodated within the normal therapy programme.

The study is important in two respects. First, it showed that compared to those on a waiting list, patients did indeed make significant progress in terms of reductions in their trauma and depression symptoms and daily living problems. These improvements were sustained at the twelve-month follow-up. The other important contribution of this study is the detailed picture it provides of a group of fifty-eight patients who had been referred to the Centre with PTSD and other needs linked to their experiences of the Troubles. The detailed overview of conflict-related trauma exposure and trauma-related disorders provided a rare insight into the impact of the conflict. For example, most patients had experienced more than one traumatic event (average of three; maximum of ten). The Troubles-related traumatic events included bombings, shootings, being taken hostage, physical assaults and riots. Three-quarters of the patient group had directly experienced a traumatic event; a quarter were witnesses; and nearly one fifth were injured in the event. The time lapsed since the original index trauma was from six months to thirty-three years. The median duration of the current episode of PTSD was 5.2 years – ranging from three months to thirty-two years.

All the patients who took part in the study had PTSD, which was an entry requirement. Nearly three-quarters had one or more additional mental health problems, including mostly depression and a range of anxiety and substance misuse disorders. Half the patient group had previously received psychological treatment for trauma-related symptoms. The research reinforced the conclusions of other studies linking adverse and direct experiences of violence associated with the Troubles with high levels of mental health problems (e.g. Muldoon et al., 2005; Dillenburger et al., 2007a, 2007b; Muldoon and Downes, 2007).

Besides demonstrating the immediate and long-term beneficial impact of trauma-focused CBT for adults who were suffering chronic PTSD as a result of civil conflict, the study demonstrated that the patients with multiple experiences of trauma and chronic PTSD (the majority of which were linked to conflict-related violence) had very significant health and social challenges as a result. Amongst other things, the study illustrated the mean number of conflict-related traumatic experiences of individuals living in the context of enduring sectarian violence and the profile of patients' mental health disorders and their severity. These findings underlined the adverse impact of the long period of violence associated with the Troubles – over thirty years.

As noted in Chapter 7, the patient group who took part in the study were typical of the wider group of 670 or so who were referred to the Centre. The findings were widely shared with key agencies in Northern Ireland.

Investigating the impact of the Troubles on the population

As described in Chapter 5, by the time of the Belfast Agreement (1998), research was revealing evidence of a distinctive and significant impact of the violence. However, a major shortcoming noted by several researchers and commentators was the absence of a population based or epidemiological study which would provide a more global picture of need – one that was representative of the total population (Daly, 1999; Deloitte and Touche, 2003). This, and the lack of progress in policy and services to address the health and well-being impacts of the years of violence, emphasised the need for further population-based research.

In 2002 the Centre commenced work on a population study. In 2003, with the assistance of the Director of the Research and Development Office at Northern Ireland's DHSSPS, the NICTT formed a research partnership with Professor Brendan Bunting and his team at the Psychology Research Institute at the University of Ulster. The NICTT-UU partnership brought together the University's research capability alongside the NICTT's clinical and community-based experience of understanding and responding to trauma-related needs linked to the violence. From 2003 to 2011 it secured a number of research grants to undertake a series of studies investigating the mental health impact of the Troubles in Northern Ireland. By early 2012 the partnership had produced four major reports into the impact of the Northern Ireland conflict on mental health (Ferry et al., 2008; Ferry et al., 2011; Bunting et al., 2012; Ferry et al., 2012). The studies were also reported in a number of peer reviewed papers (Bunting et al., 2013, Ferry et al., 2014; Ferry et al., 2015).

The chief aim of the NICTT-UU partnership was to investigate the impact of the Troubles on the adult population to inform policy, service development and practice. The studies undertaken by the partnership were based largely upon secondary analyses of the Northern Ireland Study of Health and Stress (NISHS), with additional research and analyses. The series of studies set out to investigate epidemiologically the health and well-being consequences of the years of violence from 1969 until circa 2005, which by 2006 was estimated to have resulted in 3720 deaths in a population of approximately 1.7 million (McKittrick et al., 2007).

The NISHS had been funded by Northern Ireland's health department's Research and Development Office to assess the broad mental health needs of the adult population. This study had considerable value in that it was structured as a randomly representative epidemiological study of mental health disorders in the population (with some qualifications in that, for example, people living in institutions of one kind or another, such as prisons, were not included). The NISHS was one of thirty or so identical studies undertaken across the world as part of the World Mental Health Survey Initiative (Kessler and Üstün, 2004). It involved a multi-stage, clustered area probability household sample of 4,340 adults (Ferry et al., 2008) using the Composite International Diagnostic Interview (CIDI) (Kessler and Üstün, 2004). The CIDI is 'a fully-structured research diagnostic interview designed for use by trained lay interviewers who do not have clinical experience [and which] generates diagnoses of mental disorders according to the definitions and criteria of both the ICD (International Classification of Diseases) and DSM (Diagnostic and Statistical Manual of Mental Disorders) systems' (Kessler et al., 2009: 1).

The objective of the NICTT-UU partnership was to assess the distinctive impact of the Troubles by investigating the data in the NISHS regarding the mental health and impact of conflict and related matters. The international dimension, the centralised and agreed design, and the supervision of the World Mental Health Survey studies provided a robust tool and process for undertaking population-based assessments of mental health needs. It also enabled international comparisons of trauma exposure and trauma-related disorders.

The additional analyses required to look specifically at the conflict and trauma-related evidence within the NISHS was made possible by research grants from non-governmental sources including the UK's Big Lottery Fund, The Lupina Foundation of Canada, which provided a number of grants, and The Atlantic Philanthropies. These grants allowed the NICTT-UU partnership to appoint a researcher. The combination of public and other funding illustrates the added value that philanthropic and other non-public funding can bring to public sector investments.

The population trauma studies

The secondary analysis of data from the NISHS revealed detailed findings about the level of exposure to conflict-related traumatic experiences and the associated physical and mental health impacts. Qualitative studies helped the research team to better understand the context within which individuals were living at the time of their Troubles-related traumatic experiences and the personal, family and wider social impact of these events. Later work investigated the perceptions of those who met the criteria for trauma-related disorders in relation to justice, political progress and the relative peace of the post-ceasefire period. The series of studies included the following:

- An assessment of the level and types of trauma exposure, and the association between exposure and level and types of mental health disorders (Bunting et al., 2013, Ferry et al., 2014; Ferry et al., 2015).
- The association between trauma exposure and physical health (Ferry et al., 2008; Bunting et al., 2012).
- The experiences and needs of the ageing population – undertaken because early findings suggested that the older age groups within the population had higher levels of trauma exposure and adverse mental health outcomes (Ferry et al., 2012).
- The health economic burden of post-traumatic stress disorder in Northern Ireland's population (Ferry et al., 2011).
- Help-seeking amongst respondents who met the criteria for a range of mental health disorders, including assessing delays in help-seeking (Ferry et al., 2008; Bunting et al., 2012).
- Service access and the effectiveness of services as perceived by respondents (Ferry et al., 2008; Bunting et al., 2012).
- A qualitative investigation of the experiences of respondents (Ferry et al., 2008).
- The relationship between traumatic experiences linked to conflict and perceptions on the Troubles, political progress and related matters (Ferry et al., 2012).

Findings from the population studies

The research team found that adults' levels of exposure to conflict and non-conflict-related traumatic events (60.6%) were slightly below international norms of around two thirds for developed societies (Galea et al., 2005). Nonetheless, nearly four in ten adults (39%) had been exposed to one or more conflict-related traumatic events, indicating that such events represented a significant stressor on the population. Almost a quarter (23%) of adults reported experiencing their first conflict-related traumatic event before they reached nine years, with 34% having their first such experience between ten and nineteen years. Well over half of adults had had their first traumatic experience linked to conflict by the time they reached 20 years of age (Bunting et al., 2012). These findings raised questions as to the long-term effects of traumatic experiences in early childhood and adolescence

The level of twelve-month PTSD was estimated to be 5.1%, the lifetime level was 8.8% and the conditional level (i.e. the proportion of those who, having been exposed to traumatic events subsequently met the criteria for PTSD) was 15%. The lifetime figure for PTSD provided a sense of the scale of the population impact (remembering too that there are other adverse mental health risks following traumatic experiences). The twelve-month figure provided an indication of current need and service requirements.

For the purposes of analysis, respondents were assigned to one of three sub categories: (1) those who had never had a traumatic experience; (2) those who had only had one or more non-conflict-related traumatic experiences; and (3) those who had had one or more conflict-related traumatic experience (and who may also have had one or more non-conflict-related experiences). Conflict-related traumatic events were associated with higher levels of mental health disorders, as illustrated in Figure 6. The prevalence of disorders within each of the three groups were 32.0%, 26.4% and 12.3% respectively. The level of PTSD was higher in the 'conflict' than in the 'non-conflict only' group. Alcohol and drug abuse or dependence were particularly strongly associated with conflict-related trauma exposure. The findings also revealed a significant association between ever having had a conflict or non-conflict traumatic experience and one or more chronic physical health conditions (Bunting et al., 2013).

Exposure to conflict-related traumatic events was found to be a marker for higher levels of mental ill-health and was associated with deprivation and other determinants of poorer health and well-being. There were significant differences for both men and women between the levels of PTSD associated with conflict and non-conflict-related traumatic experiences.

By comparing PTSD levels in Northern Ireland with the findings of other studies from the World Mental Health Survey it was found that Northern Ireland had the highest level of PTSD across participating countries, including

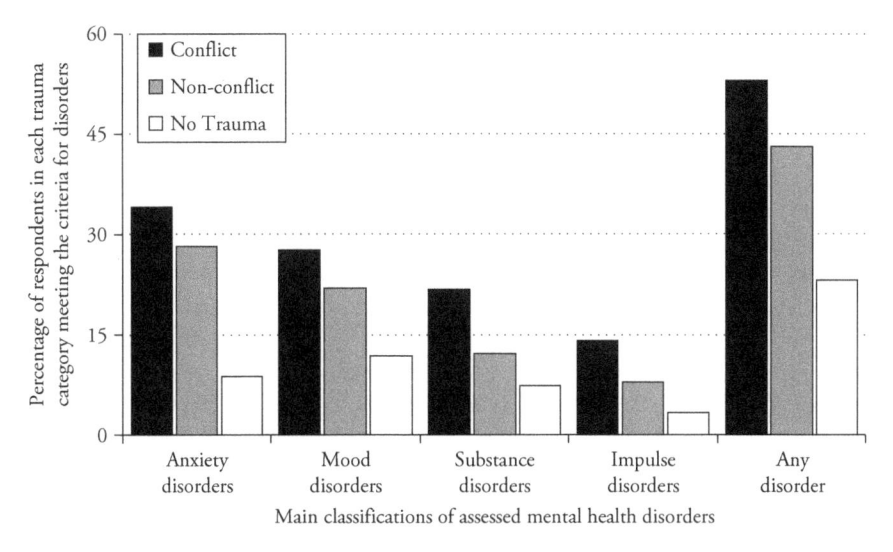

Figure 6: The prevalence of lifetime mental health disorders in the Northern Ireland Study of Health and Stress across three trauma categories

those that had experienced on-going or recent war or civil conflict (Ferry et al., 2008; Ferry et al., 2011; Karam et al., 2014).

The researchers were able to demonstrate that whereas on average people who develop the symptoms of depression seek help within twelve months of the first onset of symptoms, those with anxiety disorders take on average twenty-two years before they seek help (Bunting et al., 2012). PTSD is classified as an anxiety disorder. The findings revealed that compared with the findings of the Cost of the Troubles Study (Fay et al., 1998), which had relied upon area-based data on levels of violence, the distribution of people who had experienced conflict-related violence was, ten years later, more dispersed. Regarding help-seeking and effectiveness of services, the findings suggested that generally (with the exception of those meeting the criteria for major depressive disorder) low proportions of those affected by conflict-related violence had sought help, of whom less than half secured services they considered to be helpful (Bunting et al., 2012).

The NICTT-UU studies relied upon methods that allowed estimates relating to the total population to be made and provided a new level of evidence as to the likely impact of the Troubles. For example, the level of population exposure to traumatic events associated with violence was important new information, along with the association between exposure to conflict-related traumatic experiences and meeting the criteria for various mental health disorders. The findings in relation to population levels of PTSD showed that conflict-related traumatic events were associated with significantly higher levels of the disorder. This, along with the finding that 15% of those exposed to any traumatic event met the criteria for

PTSD, provided a calibration of the implications of the violence for the mental health of the population.

The implications of the NICTT-UU studies

The fact that almost 40% of adults had had one or more seriously distressing traumatic experience linked to conflict is a remarkable finding. It revealed that conflict-related traumatic events (i.e. those type of events associated with the Troubles) had been a major stressor on the population. The high level of exposure was probably due to the intensity of the violence in certain areas and by specific groups, the witnessing of major traumatic events by large numbers of people, and the fact that the Troubles endured over almost forty years. Within these general figures other striking results were obtained. For example, 17% of adults had witnessed someone being killed or seriously injured. Another finding revealed that men were much more likely than women to experience conflict events – 49.8% compared with 29.1%. The finding that, compared to other participating countries in the World Mental Health Survey, Northern Ireland had the highest twelve-month and lifetime PTSD levels seemed to emphasise the significance of the stress resulting from the Troubles.

Whilst Northern Ireland had comparatively higher levels of PTSD, in other countries there appeared to be higher rates of other disorders. This suggests that different contexts and cultural settings might lead to different patterns of mental health disorders (Kessler and Üstün, 2008).

Exposure to traumatic events does not necessarily mean that a person will subsequently suffer from a trauma-related mental health disorder. Overall, it was found that about 15% of those who had one or more traumatic experiences met the criteria for PTSD at some point in their lives following those experiences. Of those who had had conflict-related traumatic experiences, just over 16% met the criteria for PTSD, whereas of those who had only non-conflict-related experiences, 11.5% met the criteria (Bunting et al., 2012). This, and similar findings concerning other mental health disorders, suggests that conflict-related traumatic events are more toxic in mental health terms, mindful that other factors might also be influencing these results.

The twelve-month prevalence of a disorder provides a sense of current need and therefore an indication of service requirements. The researchers found that 5.1% of adults met the criteria for PTSD in the twelve months prior to taking part in the study. The twelve-month PTSD figure translates into about 68,000 adults in Northern Ireland (out of an adult population of 1.3 million adults), of which the researchers conservatively estimated that more than a quarter was linked to conflict-related traumatic events.

Trauma and chronic physical health conditions

Having one or more chronic physical health conditions was also strongly associated with having had one or more traumatic experiences – conflict or non-conflict-related. There are a number of possible drivers here, including: adverse lifestyles prior to traumatic experiences; changes following traumatic experiences; trauma-associated biochemical triggers causing wear and tear on physical health; and genetic predispositions to physical disorders being activated by, for example, traumatic experiences. The effect is that those who are exposed to traumatic experiences are much more likely to have either more serious mental health disorders or chronic physical health conditions or both. This has implications for services and for the social and economic contribution of persons exposed to traumatic events – especially those exposed to tragic events associated with conflict (see Scott et al., 2015).

Trauma and help-seeking

Patterns in seeking and providing help were also reported upon by the NICTT-UU partnership. The finding that it takes on average twenty-two years before people with anxiety disorders (of which PTSD is an example) seek help with their symptoms is of particular relevance in considering the timespan over which services need to be provided, and is of particular relevance to the context where enduring stressors such as war, conflict and disasters affect a population. Partly, such delays in seeking help can be attributed to the symptoms of some disorders. For example, people with PTSD are often highly avoidant of anything (including conversations – an obvious feature of seeking help and engaging in therapy) that they fear will require them to revisit and focus on their traumatic experiences. Such prospects can give rise to fears of losing control or to existential fears of dying in the process. Therefore, instead of seeking help, PTSD sufferers often use other means to manage the distress of their traumas, by for example, working harder, withdrawing from life or relying increasingly upon alcohol or drugs. Sometimes sufferers rely upon counselling or other non-trauma-focused therapeutic services to help them contain the distress or address secondary problems such as relationship difficulties. Such interventions are more likely to achieve longer-term beneficial outcomes if the therapist and the person seeking help identify the traumatic problems at the core of their difficulties, and that these are addressed or the person is referred for more specialist services (Duffy and Gillespie, 2009).

As discussed in Chapter 7, to the inherent fears associated with anxiety disorders, we can add the mistrust and uncertainties that arise out of inter-community conflict, the anxieties about the breaching of personal and family confidentiality, and secrecy about roles and jobs associated with the conflict. Such anxieties are amplified by ongoing violence, and by threats or further experiences of violence. In Northern Ireland during the Troubles, such concerns were objectively authentic, often a matter of life and death – not just for the sufferer but for their family, friends or colleagues. These contextual and legitimate reasons for being fearful reinforce the existential fears of death that are inherent in states of anxiety and distress, posing a complex and challenging task for therapists working with traumatised individuals.

Given this mix of symptoms and context-related anxieties it is hardly surprising that many people delay seeking help. The experience of the NICTT therapy programme showed that people who delayed seeking help for a long time often did so after the means they were relying upon for managing their distress no longer worked or the effort required to keep the trauma-related distress under control was overwhelming. In such circumstances people typically sought help at moments of crisis when those methods broke down, or because they had acquired other problems, such as alcohol dependency. These moments of crisis would often have prompted them, their families or their medical advisers to seek access to trauma-focused therapy.

Taking the experience of PTSD sufferers as an example, the researchers found that less than two thirds had sought help, of which two thirds felt they had received help that was 'effective or helpful'. The effect was that just over 40% of those who met the criteria for PTSD sought and received help that, in their terms, made a positive difference. The inference is that a little under 60% did not. This pattern was repeated across a range of mental health disorders.

The implications for services

These findings point to the importance of having services in place that are capable of identifying and responding appropriately to those who have trauma-related problems. The conclusions of the NICTT's experience suggests that, in communities affected by major traumatic stressors, first-point-of-contact health and related services need to be trauma-aware. This means that services and practitioners are attuned to the possibility and impact of trauma in the lives of individuals, families and community they seek to serve. It also means that services and practitioners are capable of managing conversations and problems associated with trauma and loss, within their functions and roles, and can refer individuals and families to more specialist services for assistance with trauma-related needs where these exist. Secondary and specialist services need to become more trauma-focused, developing competence in having conversations with trauma-affected individuals, families and communities, and capability in competently managing trauma-related distress and in delivering trauma-focused therapeutic services. The discussion above on the reality of fears about personal and family safety and the implications for seeking help, point to the necessity of services and practi-

Research, advocacy and policy support 163

tioners being able to observe strict codes of confidentiality and to establish and maintain trust and a sense of safety with patients, clients and service users.

Proactive case finding and screening of high risk groups within communities affected by major traumatic stressors might also be required, although there is a practical and ethical question about screening for needs for which there are insufficient or no adequate services. The experience of the NICTT therapy programme demonstrated that when people with trauma-related psychological and mental health disorders get access to trauma-focused therapeutic interventions then, predictably, they can make good progress. As the NICTT randomised controlled trial showed, the progress can be achieved to the point where symptoms are reduced to significantly below disorder levels, and to levels where the person experiences much fewer daily living problems (Duffy et al., 2007).

The health economic burden of PTSD

The investigation of the economic impact of PTSD by the NICTT-UU partnership was a direct response to the problems expressed by politicians representing the different traditions, who disagreed on common approaches to those affected by the violence linked to the Troubles. Discussed in Chapter 7, this problem expressed itself in disagreement over the legal definition of 'victims and survivors' of the Troubles. For example, some politicians argued that those involved in illegal acts in which they were injured should not have access to the same range of services as other victims of violence. One of the outcomes of this unresolved debate was delays in the development of services for civilians affected by the Troubles, compared with for example the provision made for former soldiers and police officers.

The availability of evidence provides policy-makers, funders, service commissioners and service providers with the opportunity to assess and understand the impact of the determinants of health and well-being and to take necessary steps to develop appropriate responses and solutions. In the context of conflict where politics creates roadblocks to progress, policy-makers and others can help to make progress by bringing resolved proposals, based on evidence, that overarch the political and ideological difficulties, and if necessary bring a new language to the understanding of the problems. For example, the health consequences of civil conflict can be recast as a public health priority and the implications understood in economic and social capital terms, or as a matter of social justice, rather than in terms that are tied to the language and anxieties of the conflict, and that therefore limit progress and restrict the development of appropriate services.

Soundings with politicians in Northern Ireland suggested that expressing the impact of the Troubles in economic terms might help to provide an alternative and more widely agreed basis upon which to understand the problems faced by those who had been adversely affected by their experiences of violence. A health economics approach can provide an analysis around which competing political positions can agree and act. It provides a financial measure of the impact of a health disorder or risk, expressed in direct service costs, indirect social security and related costs, and in wider quality of life costs. It can also reveal the costs of doing nothing and thereby give politicians and others charged with addressing social issues, a basis for making choices.

In 2011, the NICTT-UU partnership undertook an economic assessment of the costs of PTSD in Northern Ireland using primary data from the NISHS. This revealed that the direct service and indirect costs (such as lost productivity) associated with PTSD amounted to £173 ($266; €239) million per annum (2008 prices) with about £47 ($72; €265) million being conservatively associated with conflict-related trauma. Because this is a largely long-standing and therefore complicated trauma problem in the population, these costs are aggregating and increasing year upon year. Looked at another way, the study shows the costs of not dealing effectively with PTSD in the population – to which should be added the costs of other trauma-related disorders such as depression or alcohol dependency (Ferry et al., 2012).

Funding research

If conflict-related trauma exposure and associated health problems are to be recognised and addressed as a significant public health matter in the wake of conflict then there is clearly a role for population-focused research. Such an approach can help overcome some of the problems of scaling up research from local or group studies to population-wide assessments of need and service requirements. As Chapters 4 and 5 revealed, prior to the NICTT-UU research there was a growing body of evidence over nearly thirty years which increasingly pointed to population-level problems linked to the Troubles. Also, the experience of many service providers and practitioners was that the Troubles had had a distinctive impact on the well-being of individuals and communities. The earliest studies were variable in signalling the mental health problems linked to the Troubles. Amongst some other methodological difficulties they lacked the power and scope of population-wide and representative epidemiological studies. Also, inferring population impacts and service requirements from small-scale studies is challenging, especially where different research methods are used or samples are highly selective.

Securing funding for the NICTT-UU population research required the case to be made for the validity of the research, and in particular to demonstrate how the research would add to what was already known. Sole practitioners or small research teams seldom have access to the scale of resources to undertake representative population studies without major funding of one kind of another. If peace-makers and those concerned with health and well-being are to take concerns about the health impact of conflict seriously then public funding, possibly coupled with funding from philanthropic and supranational agencies, is an obvious source. The series of NICTT-UU studies was achieved with a combination of public, philanthropic and other independent funding.

Evidence-based policy-making on issues that are divisive remains a challenge for societies coming out of conflict, even though the violence may have ceased or reduced significantly. The use of research in policy-making is likely to be maximised if the research questions are posed by governments or participants in peace talks in an effort to understand and then develop a response to the impact of conflict. Where research is not so linked, even if public funding is involved, there is no guarantee that findings will inform policy, which will then be adopted and become realised in strategy and service development. Other actors, such as training organisations, professional bodies, service commissioners, service providers and independent funders also have the choice of using the findings from research to shape investment decisions, workforce development plans, training programmes, services design, service commissioning, service delivery and practice. Otherwise findings from research can remain ignored.

Research and advocacy in conflict-affected communities

Throughout the years of the Troubles, research into mental health problems has offered a way of calibrating the impact of the years of violence on individuals and communities. It has also offered evidence to inform the development and delivery of relevant policies, commissioning and funding arrangements, service designs, service delivery, training and practice. However, as a consequence of complex and at times profound political and ideological disagreement, with the state itself being an actor, the Troubles posed considerable challenges as a subject of research. For instance, there was potentially a problem for the state in commissioning and funding research and for researchers relying on such funding to investigate the causes and effects of conflict and violence. This included the very practical problems of reaching people and asking them important but sensitive questions, due to mistrust and anxiety about safety of participants and researchers. At different points in the Troubles, abstentionism from engaging with the state and its institutions might also have impacted upon research, resulting in distorted findings and conclusions. Such problems have been noted as a common problem in the context of war and conflict, leading to difficulties in assessing the needs of affected populations (Ford et al., 2009).

The desirability of undertaking research to better understand needs poses questions about the nature of the human problems faced by members of the community affected by violence. For example, what is the most appropriate way of understanding those health and well-being-related needs arising from violent conflict? Are they purely health problems that require only health service responses? Or are they more associated with and therefore more amenable to efforts to address the contextual and environmental conditions of conflict such as the causes and occasions of violence, identity and ideology, economic disadvantages, social or criminal justice, truth recovery, or some other response? As identified by a number of researchers and commentators referred to in Chapters 4 and 5, asking the right questions was critical to understanding the impact of the mental health impact of the Troubles. For example, evidence of changing patterns of service use in a context where services have not adapted (Tomlinson, 2007) to the needs of traumatised communities is unlikely to yield results that can be relied upon about the needs of communities. A psycho-social approach to researching the needs of conflict-affected communities, that understands wellbeing as dependent upon our inner world, the meanings and significance we give to personal experiences and social events, the environment, its stresses and challenges, and the relationships we live within – and the interactions amongst these factors – is likely to produce a more rounded picture. Within that wider research context, to understand the impacts and service requirements of individuals and communities following trauma and loss, it will be necessary to ask questions that relate to traumatic experiences, well-being and mental health.

The aims and outcomes of research itself were open to being influenced or used for particular aims or interpreted in particular ways that could be regarded as political or at least having a perspective on the conflict and the associated violence (McWhirter, 2004) – an observation that also is relevant to this book. Similar questions can arise for counsellors and clients and in the delivery of publicly funded and other services. Thompson (2007) observed that as a therapist, 'a greater understanding of the issues of the past in Northern Ireland is essential to promote a positive therapeutic alliance' (p. 27). The 'social location' of researchers (Taylor, 1988) (to which we could add service providers, therapists) drawn from a community that is in civil conflict, is at least implicitly if not explicitly an issue, meaning that the actual and perceived political, ideological, social, or religious identity or views of a researcher in a contested setting, could be a consideration. This might, for example, prevent important research questions being posed, or could give rise to questions such as 'why are you doing this research?' Or it might lead to research aims and goals that are, implicitly at least, influenced by certain values or world views. Or it might influence the words, expressions or questions used in research. Also, there is a strong case to be made for researchers to be sensitive of the context into which they are publishing the findings, conclusions and recommendations of their studies. The presentation of findings can be an issue and researchers need to consider whether or how they should be published, for example, when they are likely to inflame discord or place individuals or groups in increased danger.

Evidence alone does not guarantee better services and one of the problems facing those charged with developing services is how to make sense of different

Research, advocacy and policy support

and what appears perhaps sometimes to be contradictory evidence and competing claims. The ability of policy and service systems to make sense of research data and findings, and to intelligently use these to guide policy, service design and funding decisions is critical to moving research from the shelf into meaningful political actions, policy and service developments. Key to this is understanding and using the different kinds of evidence appropriately. Though clearly related, studies of service effectiveness are considering a different set of issues to those that examine the experience of users. For example, favourable results from a user experience survey might not reveal that services are ineffective. Conversely, services shown through research to be highly effective might not reveal negative user experiences. The power of studies is also an important consideration. Results from small sample studies based, for example, on claimants for compensation, whilst useful in themselves, cannot be used with confidence to infer what the needs are of a total and differentiated population. Research findings themselves can create their own controversies where, for example, they are thought to challenge the established positions of stakeholders and interests already operating in the field. It can be difficult for funders and policy-makers to make progress where consensus and cooperation is essential, yet where the evidence highlights the need for change and development. Such considerations are relevant for funders, policy-makers, service commissioners, service designers and providers. They are central to making progress, require key capabilities in using and interpreting research and in reaching conclusions that will support progress in identifying those in need and in providing effective and readily available services.

Understanding research findings in their context is also important. In Chapters 4 and 5 the absence of baseline data about mental health needs, in particular those relating to loss and trauma, confounded the proper interpretation of findings. In some instances comparisons with other countries in the UK, or with the Republic of Ireland, cast a new light on findings from local studies. An example of the need for perspective is given by Loughrey and Curran (1987) who cited Blaney and McKenzie's (1980) epidemiological study of problem alcohol drinking in Northern Ireland, which found lower levels of problem drinking in comparison to other areas (in the USA). However, Loughrey and Curran advised that these findings should be understood in the context of Northern Ireland's generally conservative attitudes to alcohol drinking in both of the main traditions. They concluded, therefore, that the actual drinking population might be smaller than in comparable less conservative contexts. So, whilst the number of problem drinkers formed a relatively smaller proportion of the total population, they formed a markedly greater proportion of those who use alcohol.

In a contested situation, reaching consensus on policy priorities and actions can be challenging but can be overcome where peace-makers put mechanisms in place to resolve complex and contentious matters. For example, one of the functions of Northern Ireland's independent Commission for Victims and Survivors has been to synthesise research across a number of identified areas of need, to prioritise areas for action, and to bring forward resolved policy advice (CVSNI, 2012).

Conclusions

The experience of the needs-assessments undertaken after the Omagh bombing (Chapter 3) and the NICTT research programme, including the work of the NICTT-UU partnership, points to the benefit and necessity of asking people directly about their experiences, needs and service requirements. As noted in Chapters 4 and 5, taking into account perceptions of the awareness and impact of violence and the perceptions of victimhood in relation to experiences of violence (e.g. the research by Cairns and colleagues) provides perspective. It reveals, for example, how people seemed to cope during the Troubles. Also, how those who prefer not to present themselves as victims of the conflict may still have significant health and well-being needs arising from direct experiences of violence. This points to the hidden victims, whose presence and needs should be counted when it comes to developing responses to violent conflict.

Representative population (epidemiological) research can provide an understanding of the needs of the general population that can be confidently relied upon to support policy and service development. Studies of specific communities' and groups' needs can provide more detailed insights, in support of more nuanced responses in policy, service design and delivery. Researching populations affected by violent and sectarian conflict, such as the Troubles, is fraught with a number of difficulties and sensitivities. This includes ensuring that the most appropriate methods are deployed and that the right questions are asked. Research alone does not guarantee that appropriate responses in policy and services will follow. Populations rely upon systems and processes that can intelligently interpret and translate research into meaningful policy and service developments. In the most favourable of circumstances, action often lags too far behind the publication of research. In the context of communities coming out of conflict, the challenges include the difficulties that communities and their leaders have in reaching a consensus that all can live with and upon which meaningful responses can be made.

10

Planning for and responding to the mental health impact of conflict

The preceding chapters have provided an account of the experiences of responding to the adverse mental health and well-being consequences of the Omagh bombing and other violence in Northern Ireland, and a wider review of the impact of the Troubles. This final chapter will outline some of the key conclusions, focusing on those lessons and considerations that will hopefully be of assistance in other contexts of violence and tragedy.

The problem of mental health at the peace talks

In mental health terms, perhaps the most immediate and significant contribution that politics can make is to bring violence to an end. The ending of violence, which in Northern Ireland has been a process stretched out over many years and not one specific event, reduces or brings to an end further loss and exposure to traumatic events linked to conflict. It also stops the wear and tear caused by ongoing violence to the feelings and well-being of those who previously have been bereaved and otherwise suffered. Beyond this, loss, grief and trauma, and the mental and wider health consequences of violent conflict do not fit easily into the peace-making and conflict resolution space.

As has already been discussed, the health impact of violence and conflict may provoke deep feelings about responsibility for violence and its origins, grievances over the use of violence and disagreements as to who is and who is not a 'victim'. In civil conflict, mental health and such social concerns get caught in a no-man's land created by these discomforts over the suffering of citizens at the hands of other citizens. It is therefore not surprising that such uncomfortable issues – that draw attention to rationales for and consequences of civil conflict – do not easily find a place in processes that rely for their progress on political deals. Additionally, it is hard for mental health to match the big political priorities of political interests such as: demilitarisation and the reformation of policing; the protection of the interests of those who served the state; consideration of the future of prisoners; the reintegration of activists; constitutional stability and reform; and the cultural and global justice claims of different parties. Even when viewed as a human rights issue, the health and related impact on individuals can give rise to discomforts and disagreements, in the context of a history of civil conflict. Here again, where a common perspective might open up opportunities for progress, politicians and political parties can struggle to deliver a comprehensive response to all who have suffered through violence.

Politicians have promises to keep, which in the light of unfolding politics, new realities and the passing of time, get harder to deliver upon. One such issue is that of the politically unavoidable commitment to justice and truth for victims of conflict which, with the passing of time, becomes increasingly unrealisable, and, if realised, can be a threat to the developing peace process and its institutions. Political parties have to keep faith with their electorates, and thereby maintain the possibility of re-election at the next election. In civil conflict in particular, progress is often a zero-sum phenomenon. One politician's desirable political progress can be another's setback. There are risks in conceding too much and in going beyond what memory of the conflict can support. Politically, there remains 'your' victims and 'my' victims and until politics finds ways of overarching such constraints, those affected by war and conflict run the risk of failing to benefit from the optimism and progress created by peace.

So, making peace and building it when agreements are reached, requires those involved in peace and political processes to address the consequences of the violent conflict of ideas. Political progress in Northern Ireland, uncertain but significant since the Belfast Agreement, has moved forward, working through a series of crises that have been resolved largely through political deals. This often involved parties to the negotiations getting something they could take credit for or that endorsed their world view and political and electoral aims. One area of difficulty has been progress on health and well-being related to the Troubles. For instance, in 2014, an agreement amongst political parties in Northern Ireland and the British and Irish Governments – the Stormont House Agreement (2014) – which collapsed in 2015, contained a commitment to progressing pensions for those who had been severely injured in the Troubles, and the development of specialist trauma mental health services. In the subsequent deal, the Fresh Start Agreement (2015), which sought to restart the failed Stormont House Agreement, both commitments were absent, as was a wider programme to address extensive unresolved justice-related matters linked to the years of violent conflict. Notwithstanding these difficulties, in 2016 Northern Ireland's health minister announced funding for a new mental trauma service. This development relied upon the action of a departmental minister, acting outside the formal mechanisms of interparty and intergovernmental talks, to enable progress to be made. (See more below.)

Making progress on health and well-being

It must be of utmost importance that the social and health needs of populations and individuals affected by conflict are addressed in a way that brings relief as quickly as possible and minimises the onset of long-term, complex and wider intergenerational problems. Things do not stand still, and a failure to act has consequences. For example, people's mental health problems become chronic and complicated, with, for example, increased alcohol dependency – all of which has wider social and economic implications. Progress is unlikely unless key actors and institutions recognise and understand the problems, their short- and long-term implications and the possible solutions.

Improvements in the well-being of trauma-affected communities and groups and in the numbers with trauma-related disorders are not likely to be realised solely by actions aimed at delivering on issues such as justice, acknowledgement, reparation, conflict resolution, or economic and social progress. Whilst important and often fundamentally vital, these measures do not themselves assure recovery from trauma-related disorders and mental health problems (Başoglu et al., 2005). Even if there is progress on the these issues and decisions regarding, for example, building social support, social networks and social cohesion (i.e. social capital) (Putnam, 1993) are reached, this does not necessarily work for the betterment of everyone's well-being. Murphy (2008) concludes, 'Social capital can have negative effects on psychological health and well-being, producing distress under particular circumstances. Individuals are susceptible when resources are limited, when contact with the stressor is continual and when there is pressure to conform to group norms' (p. 58).

Hearing those who have been affected by conflict

At the heart of making progress is the commitment to and the means by which those affected by violent conflict are identified, heard and responded to. This is not an easy task in the context of a civil conflict, and one in which there is more than two sides. The Troubles have shown that many affected by violence who have experienced loss, injury and trauma are hidden from public view, and those affected by violence in civil conflict often have different and even opposing views on what sort of responses should be put in place.

There is a risk that needs are defined only in terms of what services are available. It is important that those affected by violence are also enabled to identify and define their needs in their own terms and in terms relevant to a trauma-affected population. Northern Ireland's Commission for Victims and Survivors required it to establish a Victims and Survivors Forum through which resolved views on needs and service requirements could be reached, and which could be used to inform policy. This institutional dimension to listening to victims and survivors is important in formally acknowledging the place of those affected by the conflict in the emerging post-conflict community. The Forum has afforded members time and resources to ponder the experiences and needs of those affected by violence and to bring forward resolved analyses and proposals. However, it is unlikely to be sufficient, and other ways and means are needed to hear the experiences and views of the many who are not part of such formal structures. Direct evidence of need is important. Another part of the post-conflict architecture in Northern Ireland, the Victims and Survivors Service, has a key role to play in collating evidence of the daily experiences and needs of those adversely affected by violence. Likewise, the agencies with which the Service works and through which it delivers its services. More widely, audit and the collection of needs and therapy-related data by service providers and practitioners are key to this process. Publicly provided health services have a role to play in articulating the nature of the need and in finding out about how it is related, directly or indirectly, to the conflict. Research and audit are key to understanding the specific and changing needs of conflict-affected communities. The news and current affairs media in their various formats can play a role in helping the wider community to understand the enduring impact of the conflict, and in driving progress.

These endeavours will benefit from being mindful of safety and trust considerations, of cultural matters and particularly of how loss and distress are expressed and dealt with, of how the individual understands and describes his or her inner world, feelings and needs, and how he or she relates to family and community. Important too are the place of religious faith and practice in the lives of people and their communities, and the need for acknowledgement through ritual and declarations of what people have suffered, lost, endured and hope for. There is a place for traditional and new rites of passage to enable voices to be heard and ways forward to be found. The language used by people and their communities to think about and describe distress and mental health problems is an important consideration and ways need to be found to interconnect this with the more formal languages of counselling, psychology and psychiatry. The influences of stigma and superstition need to be considered, and in particular how these might act as barriers to help-seeking and the take-up of services. Finally, there is the necessity of hearing the expression of loss and grief, the possibility to think and talk about outrage, grievance, guilt, shame, injustice, forgiveness and mercy.

There is the need to be aware of those whose voices are not heard. In Northern Ireland the term 'victims and survivors' has been in common usage to describe those who are likely to need services. Yet, as research reviewed in Chapter 5 revealed, some people who were deeply affected by experiences of violence do not regard themselves as either victims or survivors in the formal sense in which the term is used. This means that if services are promoted as being for victims and survivors then those who reject this term may never hear about, or may be unable or unwilling, to access services that would otherwise be relevant to them.

Setting a destination and direction for therapeutic services

Once the impact, the need and their consequences are recognised, progress will rely upon the identification of desired outcomes and the steps required to achieve these. In this context the destination is chiefly a public health one – the well-being and resilience of a population, with particular regard for those who have been most directly affected by violence.

To deliver an effective and ethical response, policy-makers, service providers, practitioners, and so on require ways of understanding the needs of the individual in a manner that takes into account the circumstances in which they are living, their stresses and resources, and the wider social determinants of health and well-being (Marmot and Wilkinson, 2011). The approach should allow assistance to be given, confident that interventions will do no harm, have a very good chance of bringing benefit and are not wasteful of scarce resources. Properly, such interventions and their effects should be capable of being understood by, and be meaningful for, the person or family seeking help. The knowledge and skills of the person providing help should be drawn from a competent body of knowledge that is always being renewed and refined in the light of experiences, reflection and new discoveries. It is important that the person and agency delivering services are able to understand why a person seeking help benefited from the intervention they received, so that the lessons can be made available for the benefit of others. It is also important to understand why a person seeking help did not benefit, so that services and interventions can be improved. It is clearly desirable that other practitioners can acquire the same knowledge, skills and capability, so that even more people can benefit. To do these things it is necessary to rely on one or more frameworks underpinned by theory, evidence, experience and principles that provide ways of understanding needs, describing interventions and determining therapeutic goals that are meaningful to the person seeking help – and that enable them to reach a better place. It is about having a scientific and systematic approach, which provides a means of understanding the needs of an individual or the needs of a population and yet within the hands of the competent helper, researcher or policy-maker can be used flexibly with regard for the forms of expression, experiences, needs, culture, world views and recovery aims of the person (or population) concerned.

The research described in previous chapters reveals that traumatic experiences and circumstances are significant risk factors for both mental and physical health. In war and conflict, where the stressors of violence are significantly, if not overwhelmingly, traumatic – then it makes sense to consider the health and well-being risks by assessing both the levels of exposure to traumatic events and the adverse health outcomes. It follows that amongst conflict-affected populations, policies and services should be designed to approach the difficulties faced by individuals, families and communities with a focused (but not exclusive) attention to traumatic risks and experiences. This could include specific initiatives to identify those at risk through research, screening, case finding, or through special measures incorporated into everyday first-point-of-contact services. Experience in Omagh showed how relevant and useful a trauma-focused approach could be. Not only did this support the development of therapeutic services, practice and the setting of therapeutic goals, but also provided a rationale for key political, policy, managerial and governance decisions. The approach also enabled funders to understand the problems, the aims of services and the nature of the desired outcomes. Given it had relevance for the therapeutic, managerial, civic and political spheres, and acting as a unifying model or theory, the trauma-focused approach supported the interconnectivity amongst these areas of activity and created a common purpose and aim, in what might otherwise have been a disjointed response to the traumatised community.

The therapeutic endeavour itself – underpinned by effective assessment with the individual – requires an explanatory model of trauma that contains the essential features of the traumatic reaction set in a theory of why we sometimes suffer adverse psychological traumatic responses to terrible life experiences. Such a model is central to the design and delivery of services and to the aims and content of training, staff supervision and support. It should explain why we sometimes become traumatised, why unhelpful, distressing and destructive symptoms and responses to traumatic experiences are maintained (instead of being resolved), and what it takes for the person within the therapeutic relationship to address their trauma-related problems. Mindful that people have wider needs with other origins, the trauma-focused approach should be set in a wider body of knowledge of human experience and need, which incorporates the physical and emotional aspect of our being, our thinking, our existential or spiritual needs, our relationships, our strengths and deprivations, our environment, and other dimensions of life and well-being. In the context of conflict this also requires sensitivity to how we view and describe ourselves and our needs in a divided and conflicted world, and to issues of safety, justice, belonging and identity. Furthermore, the problems we seek help for might not be trauma-related – even though the traumatic experience prompted us to seek help. Careful assessment of needs at the outset and continually throughout the therapeutic engagement will enable services to determine with the person seeking help whether the presented and revealed problems require a trauma-focused response or some other approach, or both.

A narrative of trauma and recovery is critical to the contribution of leaders. Leadership that authentically and empathetically acknowledges loss, grief and trauma, draws attention to the strength and resilience of communities, and imagines that recovery and growth in time to come, is necessary for the journey that communities need to follow after conflict. In responding to individual tragedies and in looking back at the losses and traumas of recent past conflicts that are

Planning and responding   175

ending, acknowledgement and remembrance are important. At the collective and national levels these can be formalised, for example, in religious and political events. Yet acknowledgment in civil conflict can be fraught with problems in finding the balance between truthfully and authentically acknowledging something, without isolating and affronting others who have been affected by the conflict, those who have been forgotten and those who are thought of as being on the other side of the conflict.

Constructing a response for post-conflict recovery

Experience in Northern Ireland suggests interventions are required at both the collective and personal levels. The precise policies, initiatives and services will need to be determined through consultations and research with the affected communities.

Broad actions are required to address the conditions, deprivations and missed opportunities of communities and groups. This may require political, social and economic actions to address on-going violence and the sense of danger or threat, the fault lines that create factional and sectarian senses of exclusion, the economic and social deprivations and inequalities that impinge upon well-being, and the structural barriers that get in the way of people recovering, or seeking and receiving help. Such broad actions can also help orientate the contributions and actions of government and supranational aid organisations, the efforts of governmental departments, the public service sector, and the not-for-profit and private sectors so that there is a common purpose towards clearly identified goals and outcomes.

The Delivering Social Change initiative of Northern Ireland's Executive provides an example of such a programme. This was established 'to deliver a sustained reduction in poverty and associated issues across all ages and to improve children and young people's health, well-being and life opportunities, thereby breaking the long-term cycle of multi-generational problems' (Executive Office, 2016). The initiative seeks to work across government departments thereby overcoming obstacles created by interdepartmental boundaries, and to achieve social benefits through a small number of actions focused on outcomes, 'which can really make a difference to people's lives'.

Narrow actions, principally at the personal level will also be required. This should include therapeutic measures aimed at understanding and addressing the distress and functional problems faced by individuals and families – including the adverse experiences of hostility and problems of loss and trauma-related mental health disorders. Such programmes should be designed, for example, to help identify and understand those with loss and trauma-related problems, be capable of supporting people with such needs and delivering skilled and specialist services to those who need them. They must also support families, key

> **Community recovery-focused actions**
>
> Wider policy actions to reduce violence, reduce fear, address sectarianism, build confidence and cohesion, build stake holding, etc. Processes of acknowledgement.
>
> Wider community education initiatives to improve skills and knowledge in wellbeing, resilience and relationships.
>
> Addressing social and economic conditions associated with, or that exacerbate, loss, grief and trauma.
>
> Finding solutions to unresolved justice issues, and other legacies of conflict.
>
> **Individual and family-focused therapeutic actions**
>
> Develop engagement, capability and contribution of not-for-profit, community-based organisations, faith communities, employers etc.
>
> Expand and develop capability and capacity of public provided and not-for-profit psycho-social and mental health services in primary and community care settings.
>
> Expand and develop specialist trauma-focused therapeutic and associated support services. Develop capability to identify and respond to personal and family inter-generational problems.

Figure 7: Overview of possible measures to promote the capabilities of community members and key services to address the immediate and long-term impact of major traumatic stressors on individuals, families and communities

relationships, parenting and child development as such measures are central to limiting the trans-generational consequences of conflict (O'Neill et al., 2015; Pearson, 2016). These initiatives need to be as widely and routinely accessible as possible to the conflict-affected population.

As Northern Ireland illustrates, needs change over time – as violence rages and ends, and then into the post-conflict and reconstruction periods. The priorities of ordinary people who have experienced the violence of conflict at first hand need to be understood and constantly evaluated if policy, funding, services and practice are to keep pace with changes in their needs and priorities. Also, the expressed views of individuals, families and communities might be different from the priorities and perceptions of politicians and other actors. For example, a study undertaken in Northern Ireland in 2014–2015 identified the priorities amongst agencies and other respondents concerned with the trans-generational impact of the Troubles. The main categories and concerns were prioritised by respondents as follows.

- Health and well-being needs – in particular, mental ill-health and substance abuse or dependency.
- Family, parenting and relationship problems – in particular, interpersonal or family conflict, and poor family functioning.

- Life opportunities and outcomes – in particular, social isolation and solidarity needs, poor participation in education and related services, and economic hardship, debt and poverty.
- 'Dealing with the past' (i.e. addressing the outstanding justice and related legacy of the years of violence in Northern Ireland), the principal concern being the desire or search for truth, about past events. (Bolton and Devine, 2015)

At the time this study was undertaken, the political system in Northern Ireland was placing its priorities on finding ways of 'dealing with the past' (Stormont House Agreement, 2014).

In summary, constructing a service framework that can deliver on the broad and narrow actions required to address the needs of a traumatised community will support policy development, the development of the competences of services and the range of services required for a graduated and stepped care system. Bolton and Healey identified the following components of such a system as it seemed appropriate to needs and circumstances in Northern Ireland in 2006.

- *Wider community action and developmental initiatives*, aimed at addressing the social, economic and relationship problems of a divided and troubled community.
- *Advice & Information Services* specific to those affected by the conflict or generic for those affected by violence and other traumas.
- *Level 1 Befriending-membership services* intended, for example, for where a person is a member of a specific group identified as having been specifically affected by conflict. Here, the main focus is on enabling the engaged person to live effectively, to achieve a higher of level of functioning and quality of well-being.
- *Level 2 Befriending-support or non-trauma focused counselling services* aimed at those who experience specific problems and require support through difficult times, periods of treatment etc.
- *Primary & Community Care services* involving mainly family doctors and publicly provided and other publicly funded community-based services.
- *Community Mental Health Services*. This involves mainly secondary services (publicly provided and not-for-profit), which receive conflict and non-conflict related trauma referrals. Here the focus is on treating identified psychological or mental health related conditions.
- *Specialist trauma treatment services*, (i.e. third-level services) to provide specialist treatments (for adults, children, families) to address specific complex trauma-related needs; support other services; undertake research and contribute to training & development; support planning & policy. (Adapted from Bolton and Healey, 2006, p.9).

As an example of how policy can develop within such a framework, in 2016 Northern Ireland's health minister announced funding for a new 'mental trauma service' (discussed briefly above) to:

- comprehensively address the legacy of the Troubles and address unmet mental health needs;
- improve individual, family and community experiences of mental health trauma care;
- improve the psychological and social outcomes for individuals, their families and communities who have been traumatised as a result of the Troubles.

The 'service will allow for a range of interventions, meeting the spectrum of need across our community. It will involve leading edge, evidence-based treatments in line with NICE (2005) guidelines, with a focus on recovery of the individual' (DHSSPS, 2016).

Some key considerations

The necessity of ceasing future violence

Strategies for the prevention of future traumatic experiences and loss, and minimising exposure to them, are important for the recovering community. When the deaths and trauma of conflict reduce as ceasefires and peace talks take hold, then even few and isolated acts of violence and killings can have a disproportionate adverse impact compared with the major uncountable losses and traumas of the worst periods of violence. So the cessation of violence, and the prevention of future violence that is somehow linked to the past conflict, is very important, and a key role for politicians and peace-makers.

Understanding the impact

Understanding the need is key to the ambition of improving the well-being of war and conflict-affected populations. It will be necessary to calibrate service levels and requirements against changing needs – hence the benefits of research and ongoing needs-assessments. The research and work undertaken in Omagh revealed that direct and multiple exposure to traumatic events posed considerable risks for mental health. This is supported by several studies reviewed in Chapters 4 and 5. Graduated exposure (i.e. being present, being a witness, nearly being in the explosion, having no involvement) was directly associated with graduated risks of adverse mental health outcomes. Rescuers and helpers were also at a risk comparable to primary witnesses, in contrast to colleagues who were not involved in the response to the bombing. Besides proximity, those risks were associated to some extent with pre-bomb health or social problems, loss and exposure variables, post-bomb health and social problems, and, significantly, with cognitions resulting from bomb related experiences.

Paying attention to the expressed views and concerns, the preferred cultural norms, rites of passage and the potential for inspirational and innovative responses to the impact of tragedy on communities is important and should therefore be factored into plans which need to be flexible and kept under active review.

Entities such as governments are central to the task of recovery. This includes ensuring that key policy systems, institutions and services have an accurate understanding of the impact war or conflict has had. It follows, therefore, that there is appropriate competence with regard to conflict, loss and trauma – in policy-making, service design, service commissioning, service delivery and practice.

Preparing for new needs arising from conflict

Based on the practical experience of the Omagh bombing and other tragedies, along with the lessons from the research into the impact of the Troubles, it should be expected that peace time and pre-conflict systems, policies and services will be unsuitable and insufficient for the needs that emerge from protracted and intensive violent conflicts. Additional and new policies and services will almost certainly be needed. The level and type of need arising from long-lasting conflict is likely to exceed the capacity and skills of conventional services. Where resources are very low and/or the impact great, this problem is accentuated. The type and amount of problems will change over time. The experience of Northern Ireland shows that policy and services need to be developed as conflicts unfold, end and transform in the post-conflict period.

This will therefore require both the building of the capacity and capability of existing services and the development of expanded and new services. High levels of need, limited training capacities and the lead-in times for new and extended services, limited funding and other constraints will work against relying solely on the development of new services. Supporting existing services and creating new services will require workforce planning and development.

Not everyone will have the same needs and in relation to well-being and mental health some will be more serious, others less so. This points to the need for a trauma stepped-care system with pathways and protocols that enable people to get access to the services they need, and to ensure services and resources are used efficiently.

A trauma-informed and stepped-care response

As noted earlier, the significant stress and traumatic consequences of conflict require a trauma-focused response to policy-making and service development. Decisions on the types of services that are needed will benefit from well-developed guidance such as that provided by the National Institute for Health and Care Excellence (NICE, 2005) and other authorities.

Those suffering trauma-related problems will rely upon widely available first-point-of-contact services being aware of trauma-related needs, and being capable of identifying and responding appropriately to them. This means, for example, that practitioners will be able to recognise and inquire about experiences of loss and trauma relating to conflict, and be able to work effectively in their daily work and roles, with individuals who have suffered such experiences. They will also be capable of referring individuals and families to more specialist services, including where necessary specialist trauma-focused services, and supporting people as they seek help.

Frontline services can have a key role to play in navigating the sensitive and nuanced subtleties of a divided and fearful neighbourhood or group. Support services provided by existing and new service providers, the pastoral and welfare care of faith communities, employers, schools and other community organisations offer important pathways to therapeutic services and support for some people at difficult times or when they are seeking help. Wider community educational initiatives can help to mobilise community potential for responding effectively to the needs of neighbours, children, young people and group members, and open avenues for help and promote help-seeking. Arts-based services can play a key role in unlocking the frozenness experienced by some, in illuminating problems and in progressing recovery. The role of neighbours and others, sometimes acting intuitively and spontaneously, is also another important resource of support and resilience for communities. The contribution of these sectors can be augmented with training and support in relation to trauma, with effective links being forged with more specialist services.

Routinely and readily accessible specialist services are central to the delivery of highly skilled trauma-focused services for those with complicated and chronic trauma-related problems. Such services (possibly delivered by one or more centres of excellence) will help to drive the development of a trauma-informed system, a common literacy of well-being and associated skills and capabilities in recognising and managing trauma and loss-related needs. Experience in Omagh suggests that these specialist services should be open to direct contact by the public so that no obstacles are put in the way of people seeking help.

To integrate the contributions of all service levels, a unifying set of principles will be necessary, with clear pathways through a stepped-care system. This will include enabling services within the stepped-care structure to be sensitive to the conflict-related and lived realities of individuals and communities. They should have particular regard for the impact of fear and mistrust, of on-going violence or threats of violence and the strong emotions and justice concerns associated with loss and trauma arising from acts of violence.

An essential task for such systems is to address problems in help-seeking related to anxiety disorders and to the problems of mistrust and lack of confidence people have in services when they feel their lives are in peril. This system will require key links to be established with other important and relevant services so that individuals and families have access to them.

Conflict gives rise to risks of intergenerational problems. Families will need access to services capable of working with children and other generations to address current personal, family and context problems, and to build parenting skills and personal resilience. Similarly, capability in understanding the needs and dynamics of families affected by hostility, loss or trauma will bring important perspectives on the needs of individuals and their families.

Finally, wider public education and resilience-building forms another component. This might include guidance for helpful responses, efforts to boost personal, group and community capabilities and resources, and promoting adaptability and adjustment. Existing or new initiatives can be orientated to the priorities of the conflict-affected community, focusing, for example, on the concerns of parents, those at risk of addictions or suicide, or equipping people with information and skills that support recovery, constructive life choices, resilience and growth.

Integrating post-conflict responses into the wider context

Earlier, the importance of broad political, social and economic actions were noted as being an important feature of the overall response. Conflict-affected communities have other pre-existing and co-occurring needs not linked to the conflict. Integration between the conflict-focused polices and services, and the more conventional arrangements, is highly desirable. The investment in creating new services can be viewed as an investment in better services overall. In time, the learning and skills developed in addressing the conflict-related needs can bring new skills and services to the community as a whole, and in the longer term.

Policy-making and other key activities

To permit the development of a trauma stepped-care system and associated services, policy-makers, funders and service commissioners have a critical role to play in commissioning services that are demonstrably relevant to the identified needs of conflict-affected populations. Such actors will be required to have the capability and support to enable them to undertake this pivotal function, in the interests of targeting need, effectiveness, efficiency, and in securing the desired policy outcomes. Evidence-based theoretical models of trauma and loss that provide a sense of direction, along with recognisable and achievable therapeutic aims for the affected population, are central to the tasks of policy development, service commissioning, service design, service delivery and associated governance, management and practice. In terms of mental health and related needs arising from conflict it is important to review how and to what degree such measures address and improve the well-being of conflict-affected communities.

Skills and training

Practitioners working within organisations that are responding to the needs of conflict-affected and traumatised populations will require a range of skills and capabilities that reflect the place their organisation and role occupies in the trauma stepped-care system. They will also need support and supervision. Table 3 is an example of a summarised framework developed by the Northern Ireland Centre for Trauma and Transformation (NICTT) within which the competences of workers operating in key parts of the trauma stepped-care system are outlined.

Assuming the levels of need are known, including the projected needs over a number of years, an audit of existing services practitioners and skills against planned levels of service will establish what further development is needed. This will inform workforce planning, training development and funding requirements.

Supporting communities affected by on-going conflict

Where the impact of war or conflict is ongoing and overwhelming it is very hard to think and act in a way that addresses the mental health and related impacts of conflict when survival, safety and solidarity are such immediate concerns. Such was the position at various points and places throughout the Troubles. It is highly desirable that someone or some agency is thinking about and preparing for the time when it will be possible to begin to address the consequences of violent conflict. To think about, for example, the needs, the services and training that will be required, the political commitment and funding, so that, when the opportunity seems right, policies and services can be developed and put in place. Yet, even in the midst of violence, parents need support to help their children, and adults need to hold on to their morale and vigour, and to have hope that someday it will all end.

Acts of violence and outrage can give rise to revenge and reprisals. They can also open up opportunities. The reality of atrocity can temper the ardour of those who yearn for war and conflict and moderate those who support, or are indifferent to, violence. Others can be motivated to act in positive ways to bring an end to violence, to build community or support others. Community leaders, and civic and governmental bodies, can be highly challenged by such circumstances and have key roles and tasks to undertake in the context of specific and on-going violence. These tasks or themes, sometimes pulling in different directions, can include the following.

Table 3: An example of a competence framework developed by the NICTT, outlining core competences of workers operating in key parts of a trauma stepped-care system

Areas of practice/skills areas	Service level			
	First-point-of-contact services practitioners (befrienders; receptionist staff; service coordinators)	Non-specialist/advanced practitioners (family doctors; primary and secondary care workers; psychological therapy services staff; voluntary organisation workers)	Therapeutic and specialist practitioners (therapists; trauma specialists)
Relate to and interact with individuals in a meaningful and effective way	Essential	Essential	Essential
Ensure their actions support the care, protection and well-being of individuals	Essential	Essential	Essential
Be able to assess and act upon identified need, including trauma-related needs and needs arising from risk of danger, harm and abuse	To foundational level	Where relevant to non-specialist or advanced practitioner levels	To specialist level
Be able to understand and respond to the wider social and economic context within which individuals and families live	Foundational level	Where relevant to non-specialist or advanced practitioner levels	To specialist level
Be able to deploy psychological therapeutic skills and methods to address defined issues and needs within their current role	Foundational level	Where relevant to foundational or non-specialist levels	Essential
Be able to work in support of more specialist therapeutic interventions within an overall care plan for the individual or family	Foundational level	Where relevant to foundational, non-specialist or advanced practitioner levels	Essential
Be able to implement, monitor and evaluate trauma-focused therapeutic interventions within an overall therapy and care plan for the individual or family	Not required	Where relevant to advanced practitioner level	Essential

Preparing and taking action

- Preparing communities at risk of violence so that they are psychologically prepared – without being overwhelmed by fear.
- Promoting resilience capabilities in communities at risk of violence.
- Promoting solidarity – when in civil conflict, people feel more divided.
- Addressing the causes of conflict where possible, modelling alternative (if temporary) positions, that assist in progressing towards the ending of violent conflict.
- Addressing the practical problems such as water, food, shelter etc.
- Focusing on the needs of children and the vulnerable.
- Helping people to find refuge or to leave if this is required.
- Developing and extending trauma-aware services capable of supporting traumatised populations and identifying their needs.
- Developing trauma-focused specialist therapeutic services that will deliver services and inform and guide wider service and policy development.
- Researching the population impact (epidemiological research) to support the assessment of needs, service requirements and costs.
- Undertaking an audit or assessment of workforce development needs.
- Developing and delivering relevant and if possible accredited training programmes.
- Changing and implementing policy to meet the needs of the conflict-affected population.

Leadership and ritual

- Articulating loss and trauma in the life of a community.
- Advocating for and intervening on behalf of conflict-affected communities.
- Desisting from inflammatory words and actions in response to provocations and acts of violence.
- Allowing and articulating the authentic voice of outrage and protest whilst endeavouring to maintain order and civility.
- Addressing the risks of reprisals and sentiments that exacerbate divisions and sectarianism.
- Providing collective and ritualistic means of expression, whilst being cautious about prescribed and expected responses to loss.
- Modelling and enabling adjustment, adaptability and coping.
- Remembering our humanity and acknowledging acts of humanity whilst speaking out against the inhuman.
- Imagining a future without war or conflict and the struggles associated with them.
- Being cautious and careful, whilst being open to the unexpected and surprising.

- Building alliances and partnerships, and finding and articulating common purposes.

Promoting resilience and managing distress

- Acknowledging overwhelming short-term distress – whilst making accessible support available.
- Articulating expectations of coping in the short term and recovery in the longer term.
- Mobilising medium- and longer-term sources of help.
- Bringing in and legitimising external help when local services are overwhelmed.
- Promoting help-seeking on behalf of oneself or others about whom one has concerns.
- Valuing the ordinary and everyday, and maintaining routine in the midst of the extraordinary.
- Centering on what can be controlled and managed in otherwise chaotic and overwhelming circumstances.
- Finding inspiration and beauty – when such things seem to have been destroyed.
- Thinking about and planning for what needs to be done to address the personal, family and community needs arising from conflict and acts of violence.
- Securing services and funding.
- Supporting other communities affected by conflict.

Conclusions

A case has been made in this and preceding chapters for taking an approach that focuses on the traumatic experiences of populations affected by conflict. This by no means suggests that other experiences and needs are overlooked or disregarded. Rather, because war and violent conflict visit hostility, loss and trauma on populations, it is the consideration of the impact of traumatic experiences that is the key to responding appropriately and effectively to their mental health and well-being needs. As the example of Northern Ireland has demonstrated, the attrition of conflict on populations should be regarded as a significant risk, of public health proportions, for well-being, resilience and mental health. This, in turn, has adverse implications for personal, family, social and economic roles. Potentially, it also has implications for the integration of individuals and groups into the emerging post-conflict community. Concern for the well-being of populations should be viewed as part of the endeavour to minimise the prospects of disaffection and disengagement, and to promote stake-holding and belonging. Further, the trans-generational consequences of conflict on future generations is a central consideration for the long-term well-being of the population.

Postscript: the rupture of loss and trauma

> We can't relent. And soon we will be gone.
> But sooth us snow, erase our harsh mistake:
> fall snow and cover all the hurt we've done,
>
> and bless us now despite ourselves. Though none
> but we can make amends, your whisperings speak
> all lovelessness into oblivion. (Barton, 2012)

Experiences of tragic loss and overwhelming trauma divide our lives into what went before and what came thereafter. Loss, injury and trauma at the hands of others, amplified by it being in one cause or another, forces upon us conclusions and meanings that take us beyond the ordinary and the everyday. Such events can create crises in how we see ourselves, others and the world around us. The certainties of the old world are shaken or broken. Former assumptions and rules may not function as well as they used to or perhaps do not work at all. Even if we could put things back the way they were before the death or hurt that changed everything, things can never be the same again – because how we see ourselves, others and the world has fundamentally changed. To tragic loss and the distress of traumatic events is coupled the crisis of how to cope with or survive this deeply unfamiliar landscape, where friendship, faith and other consolations fail us. This is a dark night of the soul – a liminal state from where we cannot return to the past, where the future cannot be imagined and has not taken a form in which we can find comfort and hope, and where the resources we have to hand seem inadequate for the jeopardy we feel. Entering into this existential crisis and its intolerable consequences is the erosion of well-being and mental health presented in psychological problems, mental health disorders, substance misuse, addictions and wider family and social problems. These heap a new set of problems on us, with risks and consequences for us, our families and future generations.

The paradigm of loss and trauma – of altered views of oneself, others and the world, of the crisis of adjustment – can be found in the struggles of Northern Ireland in the wake of the Troubles. Collective biographies are marked by the ruptures of the many tragedies of the Troubles. The decadal conflict of the latter part of the twentieth century and the early twenty-first century acts similarly on a generational scale. Making peace has involved the struggle of thinking differently about who we are, who is the 'other' and what defines them, and living in a very different world. As conflict ends, the certainties of the pre-violence period are overturned, are no longer acceptable or function within the emerging political and social landscape. Also, the ways and means by which we survived the years of violence do not serve us well in the times when violence has ended.

The memory, consequences and narrative of hostility, tragic loss and trauma shape how we see and relate to each other. Thereafter, these can become embedded in relationships, including parent–child, partner–partner, neighbour–neighbour, employer–employee and in political and civic relationships. Finding ways in which politics and civic relationships can move forward has required the simultaneous letting go or revising of the certainties, expectations and consolations of the past, whilst carrying deep collective memories of hostility, loss and trauma, with the effort to find or construct ways of living in a changed world. In the context of the Troubles, peace-making has meant addressing the profound anxieties of one part of the community about departing a safe and secure past for a future fraught with uncertainty. Simultaneously, it has required attending to the experience of another part of the community, which saw the past as failure and who have expectations and requirements about the future. And in the context of civil conflict, those who are bereaved, injured and distressed remind wider society of the war. They, and the crisis some face in making the transition to a new world, remain to unsettle the peace, the peace-builders and those who enjoy the benefits of peace. Yet, those who have suffered can also be sources of hope and inspiration, offering an unexpected and progressive alternative to what might seem inevitable on-going conflict.

Where the mental health and related problems of neighbourhoods and wider geographical areas reach a critical mass, the capacity of communities to contain and address such needs is further depleted. Political crises, new acts of violence, and clashes over culture and justice run the risk of dragging those aiming to establish their lives back into their personal and collective traumatic turmoil. In such circumstances people can fall back on the old ways of thinking and behaving they relied upon when the war was raging – letting go of the new tentative ways that are necessary for trust and cooperation. In such conditions, social problems are likely to increase – made worse by self-imposed or externally imposed isolation and withdrawal, and cultural isolation. Here, the capacity of individuals, families and communities to adjust and recover, to regain well-being and build resilience to face future stressors, can be significantly impaired. Economic and business potential is eroded, and the quality of life overall is reduced. Individuals and families face the choice of staying or leaving, subject to the resources and alternatives open to them. As noted earlier, when the human consequences of protracted and major conflict are not satisfactorily addressed as conflict ends, victims of the violence can become victims of the peace.

Looking ahead, there may be the potential that the transmission of narratives of the past, shaped through memories of hostility, conflict, violence, trauma and loss, will negatively influence the formation of identity and attachments in the social sphere and will create or amplify perceptions of grievance, resentment, threat, fear and exclusion. Such processes and outcomes run the risk of reinforcing old patterns of segregation and sectarianism or establishing new ones. Herein lies the potential for new cycles of violence. As Northern Ireland demonstrates, even though agreements can be reached to bring conflict-linked violence to an end, habits of violence, power and control can mutate and present themselves through individuals and groups who, for example, have not endorsed the settlement; in rivalries amongst former armed groups; through vigilantism, organised crime and such like. These place new – if familiar – stresses on populations and individuals.

In the language of economics, there is also a supply side problem facing communities coming out of conflict. The evidence and experience of meeting the needs of communities and groups affected by major stressors show that conventional service structures and services are unlikely to be sufficient in terms of access, capacity and capability, to recognise and address the impact of major traumatic stressors such as the Troubles. This becomes an even greater challenge in circumstances where the impact is high and resources are low, giving rise to a catastrophic state of affairs. Again, in economic terms, the additional health burden of conflict poses a real and additional health and economic burden on the post-conflict community (O'Reilly and Stevenson, 2003; Ferry et al., 2015).

Looking to the longer term, the impact on the developing child of living in a home where one or both parents or other adults have serious mental health disorders, or addictions and related problems, poses identifiable risks for the satisfactory formation of important attachments, developmental and other life outcomes (Hanna et al., 2012; O'Neill et al., 2015). At a population level this has social and economic implications and gives rise to challenges for social sustainability. That, along with the prospect of future generations bearing the secondary personal and social effects of those who suffered adverse reactions to traumatic experiences through the Troubles, must also be a matter of concern for the community, its citizens, leaders and institutions.

In his poem 'Fall Snow' Matthew Barton (2012) calls on the falling snow to make good the failures and hurts of a broken relationship. The poet captures much of the tragedy of the unformed and broken relationships that led to and sustained the violent conflict of the Troubles, along with the yearning for a balm to sooth, erase, undo and make amends. We might imagine that such sentiments are experienced in other contexts where there have been failures in relationships, competing aspirations and violent conflict. Conflicts and war cause suffering in

Postscript: the rupture of loss and trauma

ways that are overlooked or misunderstood; or levels of suffering that are sometimes beyond empathy because we who have not suffered cannot really know what it is like. In Northern Ireland the hurts of the Troubles run deep. Historic grievance, hate and mistrust resulted in hostile thoughts, words and violent actions that led to profound and widespread experiences of injustice and of loss, injury and trauma. Many wish it could have been otherwise. In the wake of the Troubles we have a legacy of grief, resentment and hurt that in the lives of many is expressed in the desire for justice, truth, recovery or recompense, or in despair. This legacy has subsequently acted against the best interests of generations following those that experienced the Troubles at first hand. The case for attending to the extensive scale and range of risks and need, as part of the political task of making and building peace, is plain from the evidence, if we are to take seriously the human suffering and the longer-term risks to civic society and peace itself. Many of those who have borne the heat of the day need the help of those who seek to make peace and make amends, and the attentions of those who aid peace processes. Here, a case is made for addressing the mental health impact of conflict and war. It is made on humanitarian grounds, in the interests of political maturity, stability and enduring peace, for economic reasons and out of concern for the well-being, social and economic potential of future generations, as necessary for fairness and social justice, and on the grounds of hope.

Bibliography

Allen, J., Cassidy, C. and Monaghan, C. (1994) 'A community mental health team in Northern Ireland: new referrals as a result of civil disorder'. *Irish Journal of Psychological Medicine*, 11, 67–9, doi: 10.1017/S0790966700012350.
APA (1987) *Diagnostic and Statistical Manual of Mental Disorders*, 3rd edition, revised (DSM-III-R). American Psychiatric Association, Washington DC.
APA (1994) *Diagnostic and Statistical Manual of Mental Disorders*, 4th edition (DSM IV). American Psychiatric Association, Washington DC.
Appleby, J. (2005) *Independent Review of Health and Social Care Services in Northern Ireland*. The Department of Health, Social Services and Public Safety, Belfast.
Appleby, J. (2011) *Rapid Review of Northern Ireland Health and Social Care Funding Needs and the Productivity Challenge: 2011/12–2014/15*. The Department of Health, Social Services and Public Safety, Belfast.
Barker, M. E., McClean, S. I., McKenna, P. S., Reid, N. G., Strain, J. J., Thompson, K. A., Williamson, A. P. and Wright, M. E. (1988) *Diet, Lifestyle and Health in Northern Ireland*. A Report to the Health Promotion Research Trust, University of Ulster.
Barton, M. (2012) 'Fall Snow'. *Agenda – Retrospectives*, 46: 3, 90.
Başoglu, M., Livanou, M., Crnobarić, C., Franciskovic, T., Suljić, E., Durić, D. and Vranesić, M. (2005) 'Psychiatric and cognitive effects of war in former Yugoslavia: Association of Lack of Redress for Trauma and Posttraumatic Stress Reactions'. *Journal of the American Medical Association*, 294: 5 (August), 580–90.
Beck, A. T., Rush, A. J., Shaw, B. F. and Emery, G. (1979) *Cognitive Therapy of Depression*. Guilford Press, New York.
Beck, A. T., Steer, R. A. and Garbin, M. G. (1988) 'Psychometric properties of the Beck Depression Inventory: twenty-five years of evaluation'. *Clinical Psychology Review*, 8, 77–100.
Belfast Agreement, The (1998) The Stationery Office, Northern Ireland.
Bell, P., Kee, M., Loughrey, G. C., Roddy, R. J. and Curran, P. S. (1988) 'Post traumatic stress in Northern Ireland'. *Acta Psychiatrica Scandinavia*, 7, 166–9.
Bengoa, R., Stout, A., Scott, B., McAlinden, M. and Taylor, M. A. (2016) *Systems, Not Structures: Changing Health & Social Care*. Department of Health, Social Services and Public Safety, Belfast.
Birleson, P. (1981) 'The validity of depressive disorder in childhood and the development

of a self-rating scale: a research report'. *Journal of the American Academy of Child and Adolescent Psychiatry*, 22: 73–8.

Blaney, R. and McKenzie, G. (1980) 'The prevalence of problem drinking in Northern Ireland: a population study'. *Journal of Epidemiology*, 9, 159.

Bloomfield, Sir Kenneth (1998) *We Will Remember Them: The Report of the Victims Commissioner*. The Stationery Office, Northern Ireland.

Bolton, D. (1998) *Strategy and Implementation Arrangements: Meeting the Needs Arising from the Omagh Bombing of the 15th August 1998*. The Sperrin Lakeland Health & Social Care Trust, Omagh.

Bolton, D. (1999) 'The threat to belonging in Enniskillen: reflections on the Remembrance Day bombing', in Zinner, E. S. and Williams, M. B. *When A Community Weeps: Case Studies in Group Survivorship*. Brunner/Mazel, Taylor and Francis Group, Philadelphia.

Bolton, D. and Devine, B. (2015) 'A survey of organisations in Northern Ireland concerned and working with the trans-generational impact of the Troubles on children and young people', in O'Neill et al., S. (2015) *Towards a Better Future: The Transgenerational Impact of the Troubles on Mental Health*. The Commission for Victims and Survivors for Northern Ireland, Belfast.

Bolton, D. and Healey, A. (2006) 'A coordinated service network for trauma treatment and related services: a proposal for consideration'. Northern Ireland Centre for Trauma and Transformation, Omagh.

Bowcott, O. (2010) 'MoD took softer line on loyalist paramilitaries, secret files reveal'. *Guardian*, 11 October.

Breen-Smyth, M. (2012) 'The needs of individuals and their families injured as a result of the Troubles in Northern Ireland'. (Report) University of Surrey in association with Northern Visions, commissioned by WAVE Trauma Centre and funded by Northern Ireland's Office of the First and Deputy First Minister through the Community Relations Council.

Brown, M. (2009) 'Community-based psychological trauma education and treatment project: lessons learned from Nepal'. Development Media Workshop, Enniskillen, Northern Ireland.

Bunting, B. P., Ferry, F. R., Murphy, S. D., O'Neill, S. M., Leavey, G. and Bolton, D. (2012) 'Troubled consequences: a report on the mental health impact of the conflict in Northern Ireland'. Report for Commission for Victims and Survivors, Belfast.

Bunting, B. P., Ferry, F. R., Murphy, S. D., O'Neill, S. M. and Bolton, D. (2013) 'Trauma associated with civil conflict and posttraumatic stress disorder: evidence from the Northern Ireland Study of Health and Stress'. *Journal of Traumatic Stress*, 26 (February), 134–41.

Burges, C. (1999) 'Effects of Soho bomb were little compared with Omagh bomb.' Letter to Editor. *British Medical Journal*, 14: 319 (7207): 45.

Cairns, E. (1988) 'Social class, psychological wellbeing and minority status in Northern Ireland'. *The International Journal of Social Psychiatry*, 35: 3, 231–6.

Cairns, E. and Lewis, C. A. (1999) 'Collective memories, political violence and mental health in Northern Ireland'. *British Journal of Psychology*, 90, 25–33.

Cairns, E. and Wilson, R. (1984) 'The impact of political violence on mild psychiatric morbidity in Northern Ireland'. *British Journal of Psychiatry*, 145, 631–5.

Cairns, E. and Wilson, R. (1991) 'Psychological coping and political violence: Northern Ireland', in Alexander, Y. and O'Day, A. (eds) *The Irish Terrorism Experience*. Billing and Sons Ltd., Worcester.

Cairns, E. and Wilson, R. (1993) 'Stress, coping and political violence in Northern Ireland', in Wilson, J. P. and Raphael, B. (eds) *International Handbook of Traumatic Stress Syndromes*. Plenum Press, New York, 365–76.

Cairns, E., Mallet, J., Lewis, C. and Wilson, R. (2003) *Who are the Victims? Self-Assessed Victimhood and the Northern Irish Conflict*. NIO Research & Statistical Series, Report No. 7.

Campbell, J. and McCrystal, P. (2005) 'Mental health social work and the Troubles in Northern Ireland: a study of practitioner experience'. *Journal of Social Work*, 5: 2, 173–90.

Campbell, A., Cairns, E. and Mallet, J. (2004) 'Northern Ireland: The psychological impact of the Troubles'. *Journal of Aggression, Maltreatment & Trauma*, 9: 1–2, 175–84.

Capewell, E. and Pittman, S. (1998) *The Omagh Bomb Response: Report and Correspondence to the Western Education and Libraries Board*. Report by the Centre for Crisis Management & Education, Newbury.

CAWT (Cooperating and Working Together) (2008) *The CAWT Story: 2003–2008. The Legacy of the European Union INTERREG III and PEACE II Funded Cross Border Health And Social Care Projects*. CAWT, L'derry.

Clark, D. M. (2011) 'Implementing NICE guidelines for the psychological treatment of depression and anxiety disorders: the IAPT experience'. *International Review of Psychiatry*, 23: 4, 318–27.

Collins, S. and Long, A. (2003a) 'Too tired to care? The psychological effects of working with trauma'. *Journal of Psychiatric and Mental Health Nursing*, 10: 1, 17–27.

Collins, S. and Long, A. (2003b) 'Working with the psychological effects of trauma: consequences for mental health-care workers – a literature review'. *Journal of Psychiatric and Mental Health Nursing*, 10: 4, 417–24.

Collins, S. and O'Neill, B. (2001) 'When disaster strikes: responding to a major traumatic event'. *Mental Health Practice*, 5: 3, 6–7.

Curran, P. S. (1988) 'Psychiatric aspects of terrorist violence: Northern Ireland 1969–1987'. *British Journal of Psychiatry*, 153, 470–5.

Curran, P. S. and Miller, P. (2001) 'Psychiatric implications of chronic civilian strife or war: Northern Ireland'. *Advances in Psychiatric Treatment*, 7, 73–80.

Curran, P. S., Bell, P., Murray, A., Loughrey, G., Roddy, R. and Rocke, L. G. (1990) 'Psychological consequences of the Enniskillen bombing'. *British Journal of Psychiatry*, 156, 479–82.

Curtis, J. (2014) *Human Rights as War by Other Means: Peace Politics in Northern Ireland*. Philadelphia, University of Pennsylvania Press.

CVSNI (2012) *Comprehensive Needs Assessment*. The Commission for Victims and Survivors for Northern Ireland, Belfast.

Daly, O. E. (1999) 'Northern Ireland: the victims'. *British Journal of Psychiatry*, 175, 201–4.

Darby, J. and Morris, G. (1974) *Intimidation in Housing*. Community Relations Commission, Belfast.

Deloitte and Touche (2003) *Inequalities in Health And Social Care Use: The Implications for Resource Allocation in the HPSS*. Research & Development Office, Department of Health, Social Services and Public Safety, Belfast.

DHSS (1997) *Health and Wellbeing into the Next Millennium: Regional Strategy for Health and Social Wellbeing 1997–2002*. Department of Health and Social Services, Northern Ireland.

DHSS (1998) *Living with the Trauma of the Troubles*. The Stationery Office, Northern Ireland.

DHSSPS (2003) *Management of Post Traumatic Stress Disorder in Adults*. CREST, Department of Health, Social Services and Public Safety, Belfast.

DHSSPS (2007) 'Services for people with psychological trauma', in Bamford, D. and McClelland, R. (eds.) *The Bamford Report: A Strategic Framework for Adult Mental Health Services*. The Reform and Modernisation of Mental Health and Learning Disability Services Review, Department of Health, Social Services and Public Safety, Belfast.

DHSSPS (2010) 'A 10-year strategy for social work in Northern Ireland 2010–2020: a consultation document'. Department of Health, Social Services and Public Safety, Belfast.

DHSSPS (2011) *Service Framework for Mental Health and Wellbeing*. Department of Health, Social Services and Public Safety, Belfast.

DHSSPS (2016) 'Hamilton announces start of funding for new world leading mental trauma service'. Department of Health, Social Services and Public Safety, Belfast. https://www.health-ni.gov.uk/news/hamilton-announces-start-funding-new-world-leading-mental-trauma-service (accessed 31 August 2016).

Dillenburger, K., Fargas, M. and Akhonzada, R. (2006) 'Victims or survivors? The debate on victimhood in Northern Ireland'. *International Journal of the Humanities*, 3: 5, 223–32.

Dillenburger, K., Fargas, M. and Akhonzada, R. (2007a) 'Evidence-based practice: an exploration of the effectiveness of voluntary sector services for victims of community violence'. *British Journal of Social Work* (2008) 38: 8, 1630–47.

Dillenburger, K., Fargas, M. and Akhonzada, R. (2007b) *The Pave Report: An exploration of the Effectiveness of Services for Victims of the Troubles in Northern Ireland*. Queens University Belfast.

Dillenburger, K., Akhonzada, R. and Fargas, M. (2008) 'Community services for people affected by violence: an exploration and categorization'. *Journal of Social Work*, 8: 1, 7–27.

Dingley, J. (2001) 'The bombing of Omagh, 15 August 1998: the bombers, their tactics, strategy, and purpose behind the incident'. *Studies in Conflict and Terrorism*, 24: 6, 451–65.

Doherty, K. (1991) 'The Enniskillen Remembrance Day bomb: 8 November 1987.' Pastoral Care in Education, 9: 3; 29–33.

Dorahy, M. J., Shannon, C. and Maguire, C. (2007) 'The Troubles-Related Experiences Questionnaire (TREQ): a clinical and research tool for Northern Irish samples'. *The Irish Journal of Psychology*, 28: 3–4, 185–95.

Dorahy, M. J., Hamilton, G., Shannon, M., Corry, M., Elder, R., MacSherry, A. and

McRobert, G. (2008) *The Experiences and Consequences of the 'Troubles' in North and West Belfast from the Perspective of those Attending the Trauma Resource Centre*. Trauma Resource Centre, Belfast Health and Social Care Trust.

Dudley Edwards, R. (2009) *The Omagh Bombing and the Families' Pursuit of Justice*. Harvill Secker, London.

Duffy, M. (2014) 'Treating PTSD in the context of civil conflict, terrorist violence and on-going threat – cognitive therapy experiences from Northern Ireland', in Ehlers, A., Clark, D. M., Hackmann, A., McManus, F., Fennell, M. and Grey, N. (2014) *Cognitive Therapy for Posttraumatic Stress Disorder: A Therapist's Guide*. Oxford University Press, Oxford.

Duffy, M. and Gillespie, K. (2009) 'Trauma-focused cognitive therapy in the context of ongoing civil conflict and terrorist violence', in Grey, N. (ed.) *A Casebook of Cognitive Therapy for Traumatic Stress Reactions*. Routledge, London, 213–29.

Duffy, M., Gillespie, K. and Clark, D. M. (2007) 'Post-traumatic stress disorder in the context of terrorism and other civil conflict in Northern Ireland: randomised controlled trial'. *British Medical Journal*, 334, 1147.

Duffy, M., Bolton, D., Gillespie, K., Ehlers, A. and Clark, D. M. (2013) 'A community study of the psychological effects of the Omagh car bomb on adults'. *PLoS ONE*, 8: 9. e76618. doi: 10.1371/journal.pone.0076618.

Duffy, M., McDermott, M., Percy, A., Ehlers, A., Clark, D. M., Fitzgerald, D. M. and Moriarty, J. (2015) 'The effects of the Omagh bomb on adolescent mental health: a school-based study'. *BioMed Central Psychiatry*, 15: 18. doi 10.1186/s12888–015–0398–9.

Eames, R., Bradley, D., Burns, J., Carroll, L., Mackey, J., McBride, W. J., Moore, E., Porter, D., Ahtisaari, M. and Currin, B. (2009) *Report of the Consultative Group on the Past*.

Ehlers, A. and Clark, D. (2000) 'A cognitive model of posttraumatic stress disorder'. *Behaviour Research and Therapy*, 38, 319–45.

Erikson, K. T. (1986) *Everything in Its Path: Destruction of Community in the Buffalo Creek Flood*. Simon and Schuster, New York.

Executive Office (2016) Delivering Social Change – Introduction. www.executiveoffice-ni.gov.uk/articles/delivering-social-change-introduction (accessed 16 August 2016).

Fay, M. T., Morrisey, M. and Smyth, M. (1998) *Northern Ireland's Troubles: The Human Costs*. Pluto, London.

Fay, M. T., Morrissey, M., Smyth, M. and Wong, T. (1999) 'The cost of the Troubles study: report on the Northern Ireland Survey: the experience and impact of the Troubles'. INCORE, Derry/Londonderry.

Fee, E. (2008) 'Evaluation of certificate in cognitive therapy methods'. Cooperation and Working Together (CAWT).

Fee, E. and Corrigan, M. (1999) 'Omagh bombing, Sperrin Lakeland's response: a review'. Unpublished report for The Sperrin Lakeland Health and Social Care Trust, Omagh.

Ferry, F., Bolton, D., Bunting, B., Devine, B., McCann, S. and Murphy, S. (2008) 'Trauma, health and conflict in Northern Ireland: a study of the epidemiology of trauma related disorders and investigation of the impact of trauma on the individual'.

Report by Northern Ireland Centre for Trauma and Transformation and Ulster University, funded by the UK Big Lottery Fund; NICTT, Omagh.

Ferry, F., Bolton, D., Bunting, B., O'Neill, S., Murphy, S, and Devine, D. (2011) 'The economic impact of post traumatic stress disorder in Northern Ireland'. Report by Northern Ireland Centre for Trauma and Transformation and Ulster University, funded by the Lupina Foundation; NICTT, Omagh.

Ferry, F., Bolton, D., Bunting, B., O'Neill, S., Murphy, S. and Devine, D. (2012) 'Ageing, health and conflict: an investigation of the experience and health impact of 'Troubles-related' trauma among older adults in Northern Ireland'. Report by Northern Ireland Centre for Trauma and Transformation and Ulster University, funded by The Atlantic Philanthropies; NICTT, Omagh.

Ferry, F., Bunting, B., Murphy, S., O'Neill, S., Stein, D. and Koenen, K. (2014) 'Traumatic events and their relative PTSD burden in Northern Ireland: a consideration of the impact of the "Troubles"'. *Social Psychiatry and Psychiatric Epidemiology*, 49: 3, 435–46.

Ferry, F., Brady, S., Bunting, B., O'Neill, S., Murphy, S., Borooah, V. K. and Bolton, D. (2015) 'The Economic Burden of PTSD in Northern Ireland in 2008'. *Journal of Traumatic Stress*, 28: 3, 191–7.

Firth-Cozens, J. and Midgley, S. (1999) 'The wellbeing of staff following the Omagh bomb'. A report for the Sperrin Lakeland Health and Social Care Trust. Centre for Clinical Psychology and Healthcare Research, University of Northumbria.

Firth-Cozens, J., Midgley, S. and Burges, C. (1999) 'Questionnaire survey of post-traumatic stress disorder in doctors involved in the Omagh bombing'. *British Medical Journal*, 18–25, 319 (7225), 1609.

Foa, E. B., Cashman, L., Jaycox, L. and Perry, K. (1997) 'The validation of self-report measures of posttraumatic stress disorder'. The Posttraumatic Diagnostic Scale, *Psychological Assessment*, 9, 445–51.

Foa, E. B., Ehlers, A., Clark, D. M., Tolin, D. M., Orsillo, S. M. (1999) 'The Posttraumatic Cognitions Inventory (PTCI): development and validation'. *Psychological Assessment*, 11: 3, 303–14. doi: 10.1037/1040–3590.11.3.303.

Ford, N., Mills, E., Zachariah, R. and Upshur, R. (2009) 'Ethics of conducting research in conflict settings'. *Conflict and Health*, 3 (1): 7 notConfl Health. doi:10.1186/1752-1505-3-7.

Fraser, R. (1971) 'The cost of commotion: an analysis of the psychiatric sequelae of the 1969 riots'. *British Journal of Psychiatry*, 118, 257–64.

Fraser, M. (1973) *Children in Conflict*. Pelican Books; Penguin, Harmondsworth.

Fresh Start Agreement (The) (2015) Office of the First Minister and Deputy First Minister, Belfast.

Froggatt, P. (1999) 'Medicine in Ulster in relation to the great famine and "the Troubles"'. *British Medical Journal*, 19, 1636–9.

Galea, S., Nandi, A. and Vlahov, D. (2005) 'The epidemiology of post-traumatic stress disorder after disasters'. Johns Hopkins Bloomberg School of Public Health: Epidemiologic Reviews, 27, 78–91.

Gallagher, A. M. (1987) 'Psychological approaches to the Northern Ireland conflict'. *The Canadian Journal of Irish Studies*, 13: 2, 21–32.

Gibson, M. (2006) *Order from Chaos – Responding to Traumatic Incidents*; 3rd revised edition; The Policy Press; University of Bristol.

Gillespie, K., Duffy, M., Hackmann, A., Clark, D. (2002) 'Community based cognitive therapy in the treatment of post-traumatic stress disorder following the Omagh bomb'. *Behaviour Research and Therapy*, 40: 4, 345–57.

Goldberg, D. P. and Hillier, V. F. (1979) 'A scaled version of the General Health Questionnaire'. *Psychological Medicine*, 9: 1, 139–45.

Goldberg, D. and Williams, P. A. (1988) 'A user's guide to the General Health Questionnaire'. Windsor, NFER-Nelson.

Goldberg, D., McDowell, I. and Newell, C. (1996) *Measuring Health: A Guide to Rating Scales and Questionnaires*, 2nd edition. Oxford University Press, New York.

Graham, L., Parke, R. C., Paterson, M. C. and Stevenson, M. (2006) 'A study of the physical rehabilitation and psychological state of patients who sustained limb loss as a result of terrorist activity in Northern Ireland 1969–2003'. *Disability and Rehabilitation*, 28: 12, 797–801.

Graves, R. and Hodge, A. (1941) *The Long Weekend*. Faber & Faber, London.

Greenley, J. R., Gillespie, D. P. and Lindenthal, J. J. (1975) 'A race riot's effects on psychological symptoms'. *Archives of General Psychiatry*, 32, 1189–95.

Hanna, D., Dempster, M., Dyer, K., Lyons, E. and Devaney, L. (2012) 'Young people's transgenerational issues in Northern Ireland'. The Commission for Victims and Survivors for Northern Ireland, Belfast.

Hannah, M. and Leicester, G. (2006) 'The enlightened corporation: psychological literacy and the future of human resources'. International Futures Forum, Edinburgh, www.internationalfuturesforum.com.

Hayes, P. and Campbell, J. (2000) 'Dealing with post-traumatic stress disorder: the psychological sequelae of Bloody Sunday and the response of state services'. *Research on Social Work Practice*, 10: 6, 705–20.

Heenan, D. and Birrell, D. (2011) *Social Work in Northern Ireland: Conflict and Change*. Policy Press; University of Bristol.

Heskin, K. (1980) *Northern Ireland: A Psychological Analysis*. Gill and Macmillan, Dublin.

Hewitt, C. (1993) *Consequences of Political Violence*. Dartmouth Publishing, Aldershot, UK and Brookfield, VT.

Holmes, T. H. and Rahe, R. H. (1967) 'The social readjustment rating scale'. *Journal of Psychosomatic Research*, 11, 213–18.

Horowitz, M. J., Wilner, N. and Alvarez, W. (1979) 'The Impact of Event Scale: a measure of subjective stress'. *Psychometric Medicine*, 41, 209–18.

House of Commons Northern Ireland Affairs Committee (2005) 'Ways of dealing with Northern Ireland's past: interim report – victims and survivors'. Tenth Report of Session 2004–05, volume 2.

Hughes, J. (2011) 'Is Northern Ireland a "model" for conflict resolution?' London School of Economics and Political Science LSE Workshop on State Reconstruction after Civil War.

Irish Peace Centres (2010) 'Intergenerational aspects of the conflict in Northern Ireland: Experiential Learning Paper No. 2'.

Jamieson, R. and Grounds, A. (2002) *No Sense of an Ending: The Effects Of Long-Term*

Imprisonment amongst Republican Prisoners and their Families. SEESYU Press Ltd., Monaghan.

Jamieson, R., Shirlow, P. and Grounds, A. (2010) 'Ageing and social exclusion among former politically motivated prisoners in Northern Ireland'. Changing Ageing Partnership, Belfast (citied in Rolston, B. (2011) 'Review of literature on republican and loyalist ex-prisoners'. Transitional Justice Institute, University of Ulster).

Janoff-Bulman, R. (1985) 'The aftermath of victimization: rebuilding shattered assumptions', in Figley, C. (ed.) *Trauma and Its Wake: The Study of Post-Traumatic Stress Disorder.* Brunner/Mazel Psychosocial Stress Series, New York.

Jarman, N. (2004) 'From war to peace? Changing patterns of violence in Northern Ireland 1990–2003'. *Terrorism and Political Violence*, 16: 3, 420–38.

Jenkins, M. G. and McKinney, L. A. (2000) 'An analysis of the medical response to the Omagh bomb'. Department of Health, Social Services and Public Safety, Public Safety Unit, Belfast.

Kane, C. (1999) *Petals of Hope.* Omagh District Council, Omagh.

Karam, E. G., Friedman, M. J., Hill, E. D., Kessler, R. C. et al. (2014) 'Cumulative traumas and risk thresholds: 12-month PTSD in the World Mental Health (WMH) Survey'. *Depression and Anxiety*, 31, 130–42.

Kee, M., Bell, P., Loughrey, G. C. et al. (1987) 'Victims of violence: a demographic and clinical study'. *Medicine, Science and the Law*, 27, 241–47.

Kelleher, C. C. (2003) 'Mental health and "the Troubles" in Northern Ireland: implications of civil unrest for health and wellbeing'. *Journal of Epidemiology and Community Health*, 57: 7, 474–75.

Kennedy, L. (2014) 'They shoot children, don't they? Paramilitary abuse of children, 1970–2013'. The Institute of Irish Studies, Queen's University, Belfast.

Kerr, G., McCrossan, T. and Bolton, D. (2006) 'An audit of the recovery and continuing needs of those affected by the Omagh bomb: an interim report for the trustees of the Omagh Fund'. *Unpublished report*.

Kessler, R. C. and Üstün, T. B. (2004) 'The World Mental Health (WMH) Survey Initiative Version of the World Health Organization (WHO) Composite International Diagnostic Interview (CIDI)'. *International Journal of Methods in Psychiatric Research*, 13, 93–121.

Kessler, R. C. and Üstün, T. B. (2008) *The WHO World Mental Health Surveys: Global Perspectives on the Epidemiology of Mental Disorders.* Cambridge University Press, New York.

Kessler, R. C., Sonnega, A., Bromet, E., Hughes, M. and Nelson, C. B. (1995) 'Posttraumatic stress disorder in the National Comorbidity Survey'. *Archives of General Psychiatry*, 52: 12, 1048–60.

Kessler, R. C., Galea, S., Jones, R. T. and Parker, H. A. (2006) 'Mental illness and suicidality after hurricane Katrina'. Bulletin of the World Health Organization.

Kessler, R. C., Aguilar-Gaxiola, S., Alonso, J., Chatterji, S., Lee, S., and Üstün, T. B. (2009) 'The WHO World Mental Health (WMH) Surveys'. *Psychiatrie (Stuttgart, Germany)*, 6: 1, 5–9.

Klonsky, E. D. and May, A. M. (2014) 'Differentiating suicide attempters from suicide ideators: a critical frontier for suicidology research'. *Suicide and Life Threatening Behaviour*, 44: 1, 1–5. doi: 10.1111/sltb.12068.

Lawrenson, G. and Ogden, J. (2003) 'Security duties in Northern Ireland and the mental health of soldiers: prospective study'. *British Medical Journal*, 327.

Lederach, J. P. (1998) *Building Peace: Sustainable Reconciliation in Divided Societies*. United States Institute of Peace Press.

Leed, E. (1979) *No Man's Land: Combat and Identity in World War I*. Cambridge University Press, London.

Loughrey, G. C. and Curran, P. S. (1987) 'The psychopathology of civil disorder', in Dawson, A. M. and Besser, G. M. (eds) *Recent Advances in Medicine*. Churchill Livingstone, Edinburgh.

Loughrey, G. C., Curran, P. S. and Bell, P. (1993) 'Posttraumatic stress disorder and civil violence in Northern Ireland', in Wilson, J. P. and Raphael, B. (eds) *International handbook of traumatic stress syndromes*. Plenum Press, New York, pp. 377–83.

Luce, A. (1999) 'Wellbeing of social work staff following the Omagh bombing; a short report'. Report for the Sperrin Lakeland Health and Social Care Trust. Centre for Clinical Psychology and Healthcare Research, University of Northumbria.

Luce, A. and Firth-Cozens, J. (2000) 'The wellbeing of staff following the Omagh bomb: first follow-up'. Report for the Sperrin Lakeland Health and Social Care Trust. Centre for Clinical Psychology and Healthcare Research, University of Northumbria.

Luce, A. and Firth-Cozens, J. (2002) 'Effects of the Omagh bombing on medical staff working in the local NHS trust: a longitudinal survey'. *British Journal of Hospital Medicine*, 63: 1, 44–7.

Luce, A., Firth-Cozens, J., Midgley, S. and Burges, C. (2002) 'After the Omagh bomb: post-traumatic stress disorder in health service staff'. *Journal of Traumatic Stress*, 15: 1, 27–30.

Luce, A., Cording, H. and Firth-Cozens, J. (2003) 'The wellbeing of staff following the Omagh bomb: second follow-up (3 years on)'. Report for the Sperrin Lakeland Health and Social Care Trust. Centre for Clinical Psychology and Healthcare Research, The University of Northumbria.

Lyons, H. A. (1971) 'Psychiatric sequelae of the Belfast riots'. *British Journal of Psychiatry*, 118, 265–73.

Lyons, H. A. (1972) 'Depressive illness and aggression in Belfast'. *British Medical Journal*, 1, 342.

Lyons, H. A. (1979) 'Civil violence – the psychological aspects'. *Journal of Psychosomatic Research*, 23, 373.

Lyons, H. A. and Bindall, K. K. (1977) 'Attempted suicide in Belfast: a continuation of a study in a district general hospital'. *Irish Medical Journal*, 70, 322.

McConnell, P., Bebbington, P., McClelland, R. and Gillespie, K. (2002) 'Prevalence of psychiatric disorder and the need for psychiatric care in Northern Ireland'. *British Journal of Psychiatry*, 181, 214–19.

McDaniel, D. (1997) *Enniskillen – the Remembrance Sunday Bombing*. Wolfhound Press, Dublin.

McDermott, M., Duffy, M. and McGuinness, D. (2004) 'Addressing the psychological needs of children and young people in the aftermath of the Omagh bomb'. *Child Care in Practice*. 10: 2, 141–54

McDermott, M., Duffy, M., Percy, A., Fitzgerald, M. and Cole, C. (2013) 'A school based study of psychological disturbance in children following the Omagh bomb'. *Child and Adolescent Psychiatry and Mental Health*, 7: 36. doi: 10.1186/1753–2000–7–36.

McDougal, B. (2007) *Support for Victims and Survivors: Addressing the Human Legacy*. Belfast.

McGarry, J. and O'Leary, B. (1993) *The Politics of Ethnic Conflict Regulation: Case Studies of Protracted Ethnic Conflicts*. Routledge, Abingdon, Oxon.

McGarvey, B. and Collins, S. (2001) 'Can models of post-traumatic stress disorder contribute to the application of cognitive therapy by nurse therapists when dealing with individuals affected by a terrorist bombing? An overview.' *Journal of Psychiatric and Mental Health Nursing* 8, 477–87.

McKenna, Á. and Bunting, B. (2015) 'Trans-generational trauma in Northern Ireland: results from the Northern Ireland Study of Health and Stress', in O'Neill et al., *Towards a Better Future: The Transgenerational Impact of the Troubles on Mental Health*. The Commission for Victims and Survivors for Northern Ireland, Belfast.

McKittrick, D. and McVea, D. (2012) *Making Sense of the Troubles: A History of the Northern Ireland Conflict*. Viking, London.

McKittrick, D., Kelters, S., Feeny, B., Thornton, C. and McVea, D. (2007) *Lost Lives: The Stories of the Men, Women and Children Who Died as a Result of the Northern Ireland Troubles*. Updated edition, Mainstream Publishing Company, Edinburgh.

McLaren, J., and Bolton, D. (2003) 'Early Intervention Programme (EIP)'. Unpublished protocol (revised 2005), Northern Ireland Centre for Trauma and Transformation, Omagh.

McWhirter, L. (1983) 'Looking back and looking forward: an inside perspective', in Harbison, J. (ed.) *Children of the Troubles: Children in Northern Ireland*. Stranmillis College Learning Resources Unit, Belfast.

McWhirter, L. (1987) 'Psychological impact of violence in Northern Ireland: recent research findings and Issues', in Eisenberg, N. and Glasgow, D. (eds) *Recent Advances in Clinical Psychology*. Gower, London.

McWhirter, L. (1992) 'Trouble, stress and psychological disorder in Northern Ireland – a commentary'. *The Psychologist* (August), pp. 351–2.

McWhirter, L. (ed.) (2004) 'Equality and inequalities in health and social care in Northern Ireland: a statistical overview'. Northern Ireland Statistics and Research Agency (NISRA).

Maedl, A., Schauer, E., Odenwald, M. and Elbert, T. (2010) 'Psychological rehabilitation of ex-combatants in non-western, post-conflict settings', in Martz, E. (ed.) *Trauma Rehabilitation After War and Conflict: Community and Individual Perspectives*. Springer, New York.

Mallet, J. (2000) 'Poverty and health – a psychological analysis'. Unpublished PhD, Ulster University, Coleraine.

Marmot, M. and Wilkinson, R.G. (2011) *Social Determinants of Health*. Oxford University Press, Oxford.

Maryville Associates (2005) 'Review of the Northern Ireland Centre for Trauma and Transformation'. The Northern Ireland Office, Belfast.

Miller, J. (1993) 'Broken Things'. Title track of the album *Broken Things* (1999), HighTone Records.

Miller, I. S. M., McGahey, D. and Law, K. (2002) 'The otologic consequences of the Omagh bomb disaster'. *Otolaryngology – Head and Neck Surgery* 2002 Feb; 126(2): 127–8.

Miller, R., Devine, P. and Schubotz, D. (2003) 'Secondary Analysis of the 1997 and 2001 Northern Ireland Health and Social Wellbeing Surveys'. Department of Health, Social Services and Public Safety, Belfast.

Muldoon, O. and Downes, C. (2007) 'Social identification and post-traumatic symptoms in post-conflict Northern Ireland'. *British Journal of Psychiatry* 191, 146–9.

Muldoon, O., Schmid, K., Downes, C., Kremer, J. and Trew, K. (2005) *The Legacy of the Troubles: Experience of the Troubles, Mental Health and Social Attitudes*. Queen's University, Belfast.

Mullan, K. and Herron, R. et al. (1998) *An Act of Prayerful Reflection*. Omagh Churches' Forum.

Murphy, H. B. M. (1984) 'Minority status, civil strife and the major disorders: hospitalization patterns in Northern Ireland'. Unpublished manuscript.

Murphy, H. (2008) '"The Troubles", geographies of mental health in Northern Ireland and re-conceptualizing social capital'. *Critical Public Health*, 18: 1, 51–64.

Murphy, H. and Lloyd, K. (2007) 'Civil conflict in Northern Ireland and the prevalence of psychiatric disturbance across the United Kingdom: a population study using the British household panel survey and the Northern Ireland household panel survey'. *International Journal of Social Psychiatry*, 53: 5, 397–407.

NICE (2005) 'Post-traumatic stress disorder (PTSD): the management of PTSD in adults and children in primary and secondary care' (revised in 2011 and 2015). The National Institute for Health and Care Excellence, England.

NICTT (2003) 'Treatment protocol'. Unpublished protocol, Northern Ireland Centre for Trauma and Transformation, Omagh.

NISRA (2002) 'The Northern Ireland Health and Social Wellbeing Survey 2001'. Northern Ireland Statistics and Research Agency.

NISRA (2010) 'Analysis of the Commission for Victims and Survivors Module in the Northern Ireland Omnibus Survey September 2010'. Northern Ireland Statistics and Research Agency.

O'Malley, P. P. (1972) 'Attempted suicide before and after the communal violence in Belfast, August 1969: a preliminary study'. *Journal of the Irish medical Association*, 65, 109.

O'Neill, S. (2015) 'The impact of the legacy of the Troubles on suicidal behaviour', in O'Neill et al., *Towards a Better Future: The Transgenerational Impact of the Troubles on Mental Health*. The Commission for Victims and Survivors for Northern Ireland, Belfast.

O'Neill, S., Ferry, F., Murphy, S., Corry, C., Bolton, D., Devine, B., Ennis, E. and Bunting, B. (2014) 'Patterns of suicidal ideation and behaviour in Northern Ireland and associations with conflict related trauma'. *Plos ONE*, 9: 3. e91532.doi: 10.1371/journal.pone.0091532

O'Neill, S., Armour, C., Bolton, D., Bunting, B., Corry, C., Devine, B., Ennis, E., Ferry,

F., McKenna, Á., McLafferty, M. and Murphy, S. (2015) *Towards a Better Future: The Transgenerational Impact of the Troubles on Mental Health.* The Commission for Victims and Survivors for Northern Ireland, Belfast.

O'Reilly, D. and Browne, S. (2001) 'Health and Health Service Use in Northern Ireland: Social Variations: A Report from the Health and Social Wellbeing Survey 1997'. Queens University, Belfast.

O'Reilly, D. and Stevenson, M. (2003) 'Mental health in Northern Ireland: have "the Troubles" made it worse?' *Journal of Epidemiology and Community Health*, 57, 488–92.

OFMDFM (2002) *Reshape, Rebuild, Achieve.* Office of the First Minister and Deputy First Minister, Belfast.

OFMDFM (2009) *Strategy for Victims and Survivors.* The Office of the First Minister and Deputy First Minister, Belfast.

Orde, H. and Rea, D. (2016) *Bear in Mind These Dead: The Omagh Bombing and Policing.* Nicholson Bass, Newtownabbey.

Pearson, H. (2016) *The Life Project: The Extraordinary Story of Our Ordinary Lives.* Allen Lane, London.

Pittman, S. (2000) 'The Omagh bomb, August 15, 1998: An experience of disaster recovery work in Northern Ireland'. *Australian Journal of Emergency Management*, 15: 2, 24–31.

Putnam, R. D. (1993) 'The prosperous community: social capital and public life'. *American Prospect*, 13, 35–42.

Roberts, N., Kitchiner, N. J., Kenardy, J. and Bisson, J. I. (2009) 'Systematic review and meta-analysis of multiple-session early interventions following traumatic events'. *American Journal of Psychiatry*, 166, 293–301.

Rolston, B. (2011) 'Review of literature on republican and loyalist ex-prisoners'. Transitional Justice Institute, University of Ulster.

Sandy Row Community Forum (2013) *Shoulder to Shoulder Moving Forward.* Funded by the Northern Ireland Public Health Agency.

Scott, K. M., Lim, C., Al-Hamzawi, A., Alonso, J. et al. (2015) 'Association of mental disorders with subsequent chronic physical conditions'. *JAMA Psychiatry.* Published online 23 December, 2015. doi: 10.1001/jamapsychiatry.

Shirlow, P. and McEvoy, K. (2008) *Beyond the Wire: Former Prisoners and Conflict Transformation in Northern Ireland.* Pluto Press, London.

Smyth, M. (1997) 'The cost of the Troubles study'. Submission by Marie Smyth to the Northern Ireland Commission on Victims, http: //cain.ulst.ac.uk/issues/violence/cts/smyth97a.htm (accessed 31 August 2016).

Smyth, M. and Kelly, G. (1999) *Final Report: The Cost of the Troubles Study.* Belfast. www.incore.ulst.ac.uk/publications/pdf/cottreport.pdf (accessed 31 August 2013).

Smyth, M., Morrisey, M. and Hamilton, M. (2001) *Caring through the Troubles: Health and social Services in North and West Belfast.* North and West Belfast Health and Social Services Trust.

Spence, S. H. (1998) 'A measure of anxiety symptoms among children'. *Behaviour Research and Therapy*, 36, 545–66.

Stormont House Agreement, The (2014) The Northern Ireland Office.

Taylor, R. (1988) 'Social scientific research on the "Troubles" in Northern Ireland: the problem of objectivity'. *The Economic and Social Review*, 19: 2, 123–45.

Tajfel, H. (1981) *Human Groups and Social Categories*. Cambridge University Press, Cambridge.

Thompson, Á. (2007) 'Working with those affected by the "Troubles" in Northern Ireland: risk factors and vulnerability'. *Counselling Psychology Review*, 22: 3, 27–36.

Tomlinson, M. (2007) *The Trouble with Suicide: Mental Health, Suicide and the Northern Ireland Conflict: A Review of the Evidence*. Queen's University, Belfast. Published by Department of Health, Social Services and Public Safety (Northern Ireland).

Tomlinson, M. (2012) 'War, peace and suicide: the case of Northern Ireland'. *International Sociology*, 27: 4, 464–82.

Tomlinson, M. (2013) 'Dealing with suicide: how does research help?' Paper for the Northern Ireland Assembly, Knowledge Exchange Seminar Series, 11 April 2013.

Victims and Survivors (Northern Ireland) Order 2006.

Weathers, F. W., Litz, B. T., Herman, D. S., Huska, J. A. and Keane, T. M. (1993) 'The PTSD checklist (PCL): reliability, validity, and diagnostic utility'. Paper presented at the 9th Annual Conference of the ISTSS, San Antonio.

Weiss, D. S. and Marmar, C. R. (1996). The Impact of Event Scale – Revised. In J. Wilson and T. M. Keane (Eds.), *Assessing psychological trauma and PTSD* (pp. 399–411). New York: Guilford.

World Health Organization (1992) *The International Classification of Diseases and Related Health Problems* (10th Revision), ICD-10. WHO, Geneva.

Wilkinson, R.G. (2011) 'Ourselves and others – for better or worse: social vulnerability and inequality', in Marmot, M. and Wilkinson, R.G. (eds) in, *Social Determinants of Health*. Oxford University Press, Oxford, pp. 341–57.

Williams, M. B. and Nurmi, L. A. (2001) *Creating a Comprehensive Trauma Centre – Choices and Challenges*. Kluwer Academic/Plenum Publishers, New York.

Wilson, R. and Cairns, E. (1992) 'Trouble, stress and psychological disorder in Northern Ireland'. *The Psychologist*, 5: 8, 347–50.

Index

addiction 85. *See also* alcohol dependency; drug dependency
Advanced Professional Diploma in Supervisory Practice in Psychological Therapy 147
advocacy 20, 108–9, 138, 151, 165
ageing population 157
Ahern, Bertie 19
alcohol dependency 34, 77, 88–90, 95, 125, 130, 137, 158, 161–2, 164, 167, 171
Allen, J. 62, 99
armed groups 3, 5, 54, 67, 74, 96, 126, 128, 188

Bamford Review (2007) 80–1, 83
Barker, M. E. 61
Barton, Matthew 188
Beck Depression Inventory (BDI) 73, 79, 119, 122, 135, 154
Belfast/Good Friday Agreement (1998) 1, 8–9, 26, 29, 52, 64–5, 67, 74
Belfast, impact of the Troubles on 84
Belfast Trauma Advisory Panel 139
Bell, P. 60, 99
Bengoa, R. 97
bereavement 86, 169, 187
Bindall, K.K. 57
Birrell, D. 87
Blair, Tony 19
Blaney, R. 167
Bloody Sunday 70
Bloomfield, Sir Kenneth 9
 We Will Remember Them (Bloomfield Report) 9, 16, 26, 40, 52

Bolton, David 177
Bosnia 112, 139
Bradley, Denis 84
Breen-Smyth, M. 87
British Army demilitarisation 5, 54
Browne, M. 70
Buffalo Creek (US) flood (1972) 44
building peace 3
Buncrana, Co. Donegal 12, 15, 21–2, 29
Bunting, B. 155

Cairns, E. 45, 58–9, 61–2, 71, 75–7, 96, 99, 168
Campbell, J. 70, 76
Cassidy, C. 62
Centre for Anxiety Disorders and Trauma, Institute of Psychiatry, Maudsley Hospital, King's College, London 130–1
Centre for Child Care Research (Queen's University, Belfast) 47
Certificate in Cognitive Therapy Methods (CCTM) 140, 142, 145–7
Charles, Prince 19
children, impact of the Troubles on 5, 8, 12, 23, 28–9, 34–5, 41–2, 47–8, 53, 57, 61, 64, 69, 84, 91–4, 104, 138, 158, 182, 184, 187–8
Children's Anxiety Scale 47
Children's Impact of Events Scale 47
churches/church communities 5, 11, 15, 21, 24, 27–8, 35, 42, 45, 62. *See also* faith communities
civil service/servants 2, 13, 15–17, 40, 42, 153

Clark, D. M. 124
Clark, D. 32, 42, 48, 103–4, 119–20, 124, 154
Clinton, Bill 19
cognitive behavioural therapy (CBT) 27, 30, 32–3, 73, 81, 103, 111, 117–20, 135, 138–9, 143–4, 146–7, 154–5
Collins, S. 37
combatants/ex-combatants 90
Commission for Victims and Survivors for Northern Ireland (CVSNI) 86, 88–9, 91, 167–8, 171
  Comprehensive Needs Assessment (2012) 88
  Troubled Consequences Report (2012) 89
commissioning. *See* service commissioning; therapeutic services: commissioning
communality 44
Composite International Diagnostic Interview (CIDI) 156
comprehensive trauma centre 103, 109, 115, 153
Consultative Group on the Past (2009) 84–5, 91, 101
Continuity Irish Republican Army (IRA) 8
Cooperating and Working Together (CAWT) 142–3, 145
coroner 31
Cost of the Troubles Study 62–3, 75, 159
counselling 20, 23, 40, 67, 83, 86, 131, 161, 172, 177
cultural justice 169, 187
Curran, P. S. 59–60, 70, 100, 167

Daly, O. E. 62, 67–9
dealing with the past 177
Delivering Social Change initiative 175
Deloitte and Touche 99
Department of Health, Social Services and Public Safety (Northern Ireland) (DHSSPS) 9, 86, 89, 138, 155
  Framework for Mental Health and Wellbeing 86
  Living with the Trauma of the Troubles (1998) 66

Research and Development Office 156
depression 5, 34, 47, 72–3, 79, 90–1, 120, 125, 135, 154–5, 159, 164
deprivation 4, 63, 70–2, 75, 82–4, 86, 92, 94, 158, 174–5
  debt 177
  poverty 92–4, 175, 177
Derry 9, 18, 72, 75. *See also* Londonderry
Derry, Bishop of 11
Diagnostic and Statistical Manual of Mental Disorders 7, 156
Dillenburger, K. 67, 79
diplomats 2
Donegal, Co. 4, 12, 15, 21–2, 29, 46
Dorahy, M. J. 84
Downes, C. 82, 97
drug dependency 77, 85, 88–9, 95, 125, 130, 158, 161
drugs (pharmacological) 56
Duffy, Michael 43, 47–8, 56, 81

Eames, Lord Robin 84
education 34, 177, 180
  authorities 15, 28–9, 34–5, 47
  schools 5, 12, 15, 24, 27, 29, 34–5, 45, 47–8, 106, 180
  services 16, 24, 27–8, 45, 121
  teachers 5, 28, 31, 35, 48
Edwards, Dudley 31
Ehlers, A. 32, 48, 104, 119, 124
Enniskillen, Co. Fermanagh 9, 18
Enniskillen Remembrance Sunday bombing 4–6, 22, 45, 61–2
Erikson, K. T. 44
ethics/morals 128, 151, 154, 163, 173
European Union (EU)
  interreg IIIA 116, 139, 142
  Peace II 116, 139, 142
  Peace programmes 107
existential concerns 133, 161–2, 174, 186
Eye Movement Desensitisation and Reprocessing 138

faith communities 12, 16, 21, 24, 27–8, 35, 45, 121, 180
faith/pastoral care 5, 15, 19, 21, 28–9, 34, 42, 45, 172, 180, 186

Index

family doctors (general practitioners) 13–15, 23, 30, 33–4, 41, 56, 59–62, 68–9, 83, 99, 106, 121, 123, 131, 136, 177, 183
Fee, E. 146
Foa, E. B. 47
Forum for Peace and Reconciliation 56
Fraser, R. 57
Fresh Start Agreement (2015) 170
Froggatt, P. 8
funding/funders 2, 14, 16, 40, 45, 48, 51, 55, 65, 67, 83, 85, 87, 101, 103–4, 108–9, 111–13, 115–16, 118, 127, 129, 138, 142–3, 145, 150, 153, 157, 163–5, 167, 170, 174, 176, 178–9, 181–2, 185

Gallagher, A. M. 59–60, 99
General Health Questionnaire (GHQ) 42–3, 47–50, 55, 58, 61, 70–7, 79, 100
general practitioners. *See* family doctors (general practitioners)
Germany, risks of violent/accidental death 54
Gillespie, Kate 73
Goldberg, D. 47
Good Friday Agreement (1998). *See* Belfast/Good Friday Agreement (1998)
Goražde, Bosnia 139
Graves, R. 98
Greenley, J. R. 59
grief 5–6, 28, 97, 107, 169, 172, 174, 189
Grounds, A. 74

Hanna, D. 92
Hayes, P. 70
Healey, A. 177
Health Service Executive 143
Heenan, D. 87
Heskin, K. 61
Hewitt, C. 54
Hodge, A. 98
hope 2–5, 13, 25–6, 101, 151, 172, 182, 186–7, 189. *See also* Petals of Hope project

House of Commons Northern Ireland Affairs Committee 56
humanitarian relief 108–9, 113
Hurricane Katrina disaster, New Orleans 60

Impact of Events Scale Revised 73
Improving Access to Psychological Therapies Initiative 120
Indian Ocean tsunami (2004) 139–40
inter-generational trauma 2, 91–3, 150, 171, 175–6, 181, 185
International Classification of Diseases 156
International Statistical Classification of Diseases and Related Health Problems 72
Irish Peace Centres 91
Irish Republican Army (IRA) 98
Italy, risks of violent/accidental death 54

Jamieson, R. 73–4
Jarman, N. 54, 74
justice 3, 78, 80, 88, 91, 93, 101, 123, 157, 166, 169–71, 174, 177, 180, 187, 189

Kane, Carole 22
Kelleher, C. C. 75
Kennedy, L. 55, 74
Kessler, R. C. 50, 60
King's College London, Institute of Psychiatry 154
Knights of Malta 16

leadership 174, 184
Leed, E. 97
Living with the Trauma of the Troubles (DHSS, 1998) 26, 66
Lloyd, K. 71
Londonderry 9, 18, 72, 75. *See also* Derry
Long, A. 37
Lost Lives 69
Loughrey, G. C. 55, 59, 100, 167
Lyons, H. A. 57

Madrid 4, 12, 22, 29
Mallet, J. 76

Mater Hospital Belfast 70
McAleese, Mary 19
McConnell, P. 72, 75
McDaniel, D. 4
McDermott, M. 47
McKenzie, G. 167
McKittrick, D. 53
McWhirter, L. 60
media, the 4, 10, 15, 17, 19, 22–4, 26, 30–1, 37, 44, 54, 172
mental health
　anxiety disorders 31, 41, 47, 54, 71–2, 84, 88–9, 91, 95, 101, 114, 120, 122–3, 125, 130–2, 155, 159, 161–2, 180
　mood disorders 57, 88, 95, 122, 134
　risks 13, 19, 24, 32, 42–3, 45, 48, 51, 61, 66, 76, 125, 129, 141, 158, 173–4, 178, 183
　services 2, 13–17, 25, 27, 30, 33, 57, 60, 66, 69–70, 80, 85–6, 104, 106, 119, 121, 131, 170, 177
　studies 56–64, 66
Methodist Church 11
　president of 11
Miller, P. 70–1
Monaghan, C. 62
Mowlam, Dr Marjorie 1, 8–9
Muldoon, O. 61, 76, 82–3, 97
Murphy, H. 59, 71, 99, 171

National Institute for Health and Care Excellence (NICE) 80, 89, 120, 138, 178–9
National Training Awards 145
needs-assessments 12–20, 23–7, 30–4, 38–51, 56, 88, 104–6, 111, 151–2, 168, 174, 178, 184. *See also* research
neighbours 5, 19, 30, 34, 64, 180, 187
Nepal 140, 145
non-state armed groups 5, 54, 67, 96, 126, 128
Northern Ireland Centre for Trauma and Transformation (NICTT) 20, 81–3, 103–17, 119, 135, 138, 146–7, 153–5, 162–3, 168, 182–3
　NICTT Trust 109–11

NICTT-UU [University of Ulster] partnership 76, 82–3, 89, 93–4, 100, 125, 155–7, 159–61, 163–5, 168
Northern Ireland Health and Social Wellbeing Survey 70–1, 74
Northern Ireland Household Panel Survey 71
Northern Ireland Office 15
Northern Ireland Statistics and Research Agency 53
　Omnibus Survey (2010) 53
Northern Ireland Study of Health and Stress (NISHS) 83, 93–5, 156–7, 159, 164
not-for-profit organisations 2, 10–11, 14–17, 20, 23–5, 27, 33–5, 41, 45–6, 64–5, 67, 69, 78–80, 89, 92–3, 103–4, 106, 109, 112, 115–16, 121, 143–5, 175, 177
Nurmi, L. A. 108–9, 115, 153

occupational health. *See* staff care (occupational health)
Office of the First Minister and Deputy First Minister 87
Omagh Adult Community Study 24
Omagh bombing (1998)
　bereaved, the 30–1, 40, 42, 46
　ceremonial/arts-based responses 21–2
　civil legal action 31
　commemoration service 22
　communications 10
　community leaders 18
　community response 8–24, 28–31, 106
　economic impact 5
　education 15, 28–9
　employers' response 28–9, 34
　family-health consequences 5
　fatalities 8, 10–11, 18
　first anniversary 17, 34
　flowers (as tribute) 19–20
　funerals 21, 23, 29
　impact on adolescents 34–5, 42, 47–8
　impact on adults 8, 12, 23, 42–5, 48, 52, 104
　impact on children 8, 12, 23, 34–5, 42, 47–8, 52, 104
　injured by 8, 12, 18, 31, 36, 73

Index

inquests relating to 24, 31
mental-health impact 39
mortuary 10–11
multiagency response centre 14
needs-assessments 12–20, 23–7, 30–4, 38–51, 105–6, 111, 151–2
Omagh Fund 16, 20, 29, 45, 105, 113, 135
perceptions of 4
political response 6, 13, 15–17, 19, 23–4, 29, 36, 106
psychological impact 43
questionnaires relating to 42–9, 152
Republic of Ireland response 10, 15, 20
response strategy 12–20, 23–9, 104, 117
security/policing issues 23, 31
social consequences 5
studies into 72
video footage 23
witnesses of 42–3, 47, 49. *See also* trauma: exposure to
Omagh Churches' Forum 21, 28
Omagh Community Trauma and Recovery Team 14, 17, 20, 25–38, 41, 46–7, 73, 100, 103–4, 106, 109–10, 112, 115, 117, 119, 121, 125, 129, 135, 152–3
Omagh, Co. Tyrone
  bomb scares 36, 41
  health and social care staff 37, 49–50, 52, 73, 80–1, 87, 103, 106, 111, 113, 115–16, 123, 127, 129, 132, 136, 139, 144, 146, 183. *See also* staff care (occupational health)
  Market Street 8, 12
  Tara Centre 14
Omagh District Council 10, 16, 29, 107
  chief executive 11, 29
  leisure centre 10–11, 18
Omagh Support and Self-Help Group 31
O'Malley, P. P. 57
O'Neill, S. 94–5
O'Reilly, D. 70, 74–5
Oxford University 32

parents/parenting 34–5, 47–8, 91–4, 117, 176, 181–2, 187–8

peace-making/peace-building 2, 65, 107, 128, 164, 167, 169–70, 178, 187, 189
Personal Experience and Impact of the Troubles Questionnaire 79
Petals of Hope project 22, 110
physical health (impaired)/chronic conditions 5, 42, 49–50, 53, 61, 64, 66, 75, 82–3, 86–90, 125, 133, 157–8, 161, 171, 173–4
Pokhara, Nepal 140
police family liaison services 23, 33
politics 6, 13, 23, 36, 65, 90, 97, 106, 113, 126, 137, 163–4, 166, 169–70, 175–6, 178
post-traumatic growth 7, 60, 149, 174, 181
post-traumatic resilience 104, 150, 173–4, 180–1, 184–5, 187
post-traumatic stress disorder (PTSD) 3, 7, 30, 32–4, 41, 43–4, 47–50, 55, 59–61, 63, 67–8, 70, 73, 77, 79, 81–4, 86, 88, 99–101, 104, 109, 112, 119–20, 123, 125–6, 134–6, 138–9, 141, 154–5, 157–64
  acuity 152
  economic burden of 2, 92, 136, 149, 157, 161, 171
  Post-Trauma Cognitions Inventor 42
  Post-Traumatic Stress Diagnostic Scale (PDS) 42–3, 48, 73, 79, 88, 119, 122, 135, 154
  Post-Traumatic Stress Disorder Checklist 77
  Post-Traumatic Stress Disorder Symptom Scale 43, 49
  scales 30, 42, 47, 49, 73, 79, 88, 152, 154
practitioners 1–2, 7, 9–10, 16, 27, 31–3, 41, 46, 51, 55, 67, 77, 84, 87, 89, 91, 93, 96, 100, 106, 112, 115, 117–18, 120, 123, 127, 136–53, 162, 164, 172–3, 180, 182–3
prisoners/ex-prisoners 67, 69, 73–4, 169
Professional Diploma in Trauma-focused Cognitive Behavioural Therapy 146
psychiatric morbidity rates 60, 71, 74
public health 20, 74, 85, 128, 148, 163–4, 173, 185

Public Health Agency 90, 114
  Research and Development Office 114, 155–6

Qualification and Credits Framework (QCF) 143–4, 146–7

randomised controlled trial 81, 111, 124, 135, 154, 163
Real IRA (Irish Republican Army) 8
Red Cross 16
rehabilitation 17–18, 27
reparation 3, 107, 171
research 27, 120, 135, 151, 154–60, 164–8, 172–5, 177–8, 184
  funding 153, 156–7, 164–5, 167
resilience 35, 104, 150, 173–4, 180–1, 184–5, 187
rites of passage 21, 172, 179
Rolston, B. 74

Samaritans, the 14, 66
Sandy Row Community Forum 90
Shoulder to Shoulder Moving Forward (2013) 90
Sarajevo, Bosnia 139
self-help groups 2, 31, 42, 65, 67–8, 97
  Omagh Support and Self-Help Group 31
Self Rating Depression Scale for Children 47
service commissioning 51, 65, 67, 70, 101, 105, 115, 165, 179, 181
Shirlow, P. 74
Smyth, M. 64
social determinants of health/well-being 75–6, 83, 97, 158, 163, 173. *See also* Northern Ireland Health and Social Wellbeing Survey
social justice 101, 163, 189
Social Services Boards 143
Southern Health Board 143
Special European Union Programmes Body 55
Sperrin Lakeland Health and Social Care Trust 10–11, 14, 16–19, 23, 25–7, 31–3, 35, 40–2, 45–7, 49–51, 103–7, 111, 153

emergency plans 14–15
mental health services 33
psychological support service 15
trauma-focused response 32
spirituality/religious faith 45, 172, 175
Sri Lanka 112, 139–40
staff care (occupational health) 18–19, 33, 36–7, 39, 42, 49–50, 76, 178
Stevenson, M. 74–5
Stormont House Agreement (2014) 170, 177
Strategy for Victims and Survivors (2009) 86
Stressful Life Events Scale 79
suicide 57, 60, 85, 90–1, 93–5, 181

Tajfel, H. 30, 71
Tara Centre, Omagh 14
terrorism/acts of violence 2, 54, 59, 70, 96, 114, 121, 128, 132, 178, 180, 182, 184–5, 187
therapeutic services
  accessibility 48, 66, 79–80, 85, 90, 105, 122, 126–8, 130, 157, 172
  arts-based 180
  commissioning 142, 165, 167, 179, 181
  design/development 25, 42, 48, 66, 70, 77–8, 80–1, 83, 85, 87, 89, 92, 99, 101, 103, 105–6, 108–10, 112, 114, 116–19, 123, 141, 163, 165, 167–8, 173, 175, 177, 179, 181–2, 184
  funding 14, 40, 45, 55, 83, 101, 104, 109, 111, 113, 115–16, 127, 129, 145, 150, 153, 156–7, 163, 165, 167, 170, 174, 181
  goals 7, 32–3, 36, 100, 120, 126, 132–3, 135, 148, 173–5
  protocols 129
  providers 73, 91–2, 101
therapy 32–3, 35–7, 41, 43–4, 46
  accessibility 154
  audit/evaluation 27, 33, 70, 73, 104, 109–10, 120, 134–5, 153, 172, 182, 184
  early intervention 31–2, 129, 141
  goals 51, 124–8, 132
  protocols 131
  safety in 131–3, 148, 163, 172

stepped care 81, 89, 141, 177, 179–82
trauma-focused 15, 20, 27, 30–3, 42–4, 46, 48, 51, 73, 78, 81, 89, 103–5, 107–13, 115, 117–20, 123, 134–5, 137–42, 147–9, 154–5, 161–3, 174, 177, 179–80, 183–4
  threats, impact of 121, 132
  trust in 98, 131–3, 148, 163, 172
Tomlinson, M. 94, 99
training 67, 80–1, 83, 108, 112–13, 115, 138–50, 153, 165, 174, 177, 179, 182
  academic 112, 140, 143–4
  advocacy 138
  evaluation 145
  skills 118, 139–48
  trauma-focused 147
  vocational 143–4
trans-generational trauma. *See* inter-generational trauma
trauma
  exposure to 19, 25, 40, 42–3, 47–8, 51, 55, 62, 72, 77, 81–4, 92–3, 95, 99–100, 136, 141, 149, 154, 156–60, 164, 169, 173, 178
  help-seeking 7, 27, 30, 32, 35–6, 39, 41, 80–1, 84, 89, 98, 100, 103–4, 117, 122, 124, 130–3, 136–7, 148, 153, 157, 159, 161–2, 172–5, 180, 185
  late help-seeking 89, 137
  latency 81, 101
  liminality 3, 186
  mental/physical-health impact of 26, 53, 56, 65, 73, 81, 83, 89–90, 125, 127, 157–8, 161, 173
  numbing 123, 131
  recovery from/growth 2, 5, 7, 13, 23, 25, 30, 33, 37, 52, 60, 66, 89, 101, 106, 115, 119–20, 130, 149, 152, 171, 173–5, 178–81, 185, 189
  social/cultural isolation arising from 23, 86, 88, 90, 133, 177, 187
Trauma Advisory Panels 67
trauma-informed response/system 7, 179–80
Trauma Resource Centre, Belfast 84
Trinity College, Dublin 47
Troubles-Related Experiences Questionnaire 84

Troubles, the
  Cost of the Troubles Study (1998) 62–3, 75, 159
  impact of 26, 40, 52–102, 105–6, 109, 111, 118, 120, 127, 154–66, 168–74, 176, 178–9, 182
truth 93, 166, 170, 177, 189
Turner, Juliet 21
  'Broken Things' 21
Tyrone Constitution 22
Tyrone County Hospital 9, 15, 20

Ulster Herald 22
University of Northumbria 49
University of Ulster (UU) 83, 112, 139, 155. *See also* Northern Ireland Centre for Trauma and Transformation (NICTT): NICTT-UU [University of Ulster] partnership
  Psychology Research Institute 83, 155
Uruguay, risks of violent/accidental death 54

victim and survivor support groups 67
victims/survivors, definition of 75–6, 126, 163, 172
Victims and Survivors Commission of Northern Ireland 53, 63–5, 82
  interim report (2007) 82–3
  We Will Remember Them (1998) 15–16, 26, 40, 52, 107, 109
Victims and Survivors Forum 86, 171–2
Victims and Survivors Service 86, 88–9, 114, 172
Victims Liaison Unit 16, 107
Victim Support Northern Ireland 14

WAVE Trauma Centre, Belfast 87
Western Health and Social Services Board 16, 107
Western Health Board 143
Who are the victims? (Cairns et al., 2003) 75–6
Williams, M. B. 108–9, 115, 153
Wilson, R. 45, 58–9, 61–2
World Mental Health Survey 83, 156, 158, 160